PENGUIN HANDBOOKS

POTPOURRIS AND OTHER FRAGRANT DELIGHTS

Jacqueline Hériteau was General Editor of the authoritative 16-volume *Good Housekeeping Illustrated Encyclopedia of Gardening*. She has written two cookbooks, *How to Grow and Cook It Book* and *Oriental Cooking: the Fast Wok Way*, and has contributed articles to *House Beautiful*, *House and Garden*, *Better Homes and Gardens* and *The New York Times*.

Jacqueline Hériteau collected her many recipes for potpourris from aunts and cousins in her native France, from friends and neighbours during long visits to Canada, Sweden, Vermont and Cape Cod, and from the old manuscripts and herbals and stillroom books of Elizabethan England.

Jean Harding

225- 1078

Jacqueline Hériteau

Potpourris

and Other
Fragrant Delights

Illustrations by Bill Goldsmith

PENGUIN BOOKS

Penguin Books Ltd, Harmondsworth, Middlesex, England
Penguin Books, 625 Madison Avenue, New York, New York 10022, U.S.A.
Penguin Books Australia Ltd, Ringwood, Victoria, Australia
Penguin Books Canada Ltd, 2801 John Street, Markham, Ontario, Canada L3R 1B4
Penguin Books (N.Z.) Ltd, 182–190 Wairau Road, Auckland 10, New Zealand

—

First published in the U.S.A. by Simon & Schuster 1973
This revised edition first published in Great Britain
by Lutterworth Press 1975
Published in Penguin Books 1978
Reprinted 1979, 1980, 1982, 1983

—

—

Made and printed in Great Britain by
Richard Clay (The Chaucer Press) Ltd,
Bungay, Suffolk
Set in Monotype Garamond

To
Madeleine Hériteau, *ma petite mère,*
in memory of summer
and the garden and the sea

CONTENTS

ACKNOWLEDGEMENTS

FOR research assistance, for recipes, for the translation from ancient to modern terms, and for the testing of recipes old and new, I am indebted to many gardening friends, in particular to Linda Huntington for her valiant research job and to my Parisian niece, Sylvie Nat; to Sally Larkin Erath, Paul and Jane Larkin, Francesca Bosetti Morris, Peg Perry, and Dorothy Chamberlain of the *Good Housekeeping Illustrated Encyclopedia of Gardening*; to Elvin McDonald, Garden Editor of *House Beautiful*; to Lawrence V. Power, Garden Editor of *American Home Magazine*; and to Miss Frances Phipps for her story of the George IV coronation. Gratitude is expressed to the Horticultural Society of New York, who made their library available; to the Herbary and Potpourri Shop in Orleans, Massachusetts; to Aphrodesia Products, Inc., and the Kiel Pharmacy, Inc., in New York City. My warmest thanks go also to Helen Van Pelt Wilson, the editor who wanted a book all about potpourri and sweet scents to make from garden flowers.

For special assistance with the British edition my thanks, and those of my British publishers, are due to Mr Ian Thomas and the staff of Culpeper Limited of London, who advised on supplies; and to Robert Jackson & Co. Ltd, Candle Makers Supplies, and G. Baldwin & Co., all of London.

AUTHOR'S NOTE

BECAUSE the ability to detect scent, and the individual response to scent, is a very personal thing, no potpourri recipe could be exactly right for everyone. In this book I have indicated groupings and scales of fragrances that have distinctive characteristics. Each potpourri-maker should feel free to heighten these or tone them down according to personal preference. The strength and quality of essential oils will vary; so will the fragrance of herbs and flowers, for each harvest is different, affected by soil, sun, rainfall and ripeness. Like gardening and cooking, potpourri-making is a highly individual enterprise, and no two potpourris you create will ever be exact duplicates. Work slowly, testing as you go, and work to please yourself.

There is a note about proportions and equivalent measurements on pp. 35–6, to help when you are making up your own potpourris or working from antique recipes. The cup I used when measuring out flowers, herbs, salt and so on for my own recipes is a breakfast cup which will hold 225 millilitres (8 fluid ounces or $\frac{2}{5}$ pint). The spoons that I used for measuring herbs, spices, etc., are slightly smaller than British Standard teaspoons and tablespoons (which hold about 15 per cent more than mine), so use a scant spoonful, loosely packed and severely levelled off. Chemists sell a cheap 5-millilitre measuring spoon, which is useful for essential oils. Fragrant petals for moist potpourris (Chapter 3) are partially dried before they are measured (p. 28); herb leaves are usually completely dried. All the ingredients for dry potpourris (Chapter 4) are measured *after* drying.

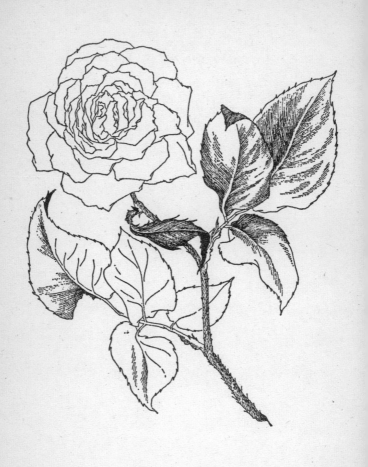

I
The Fragrant Centuries

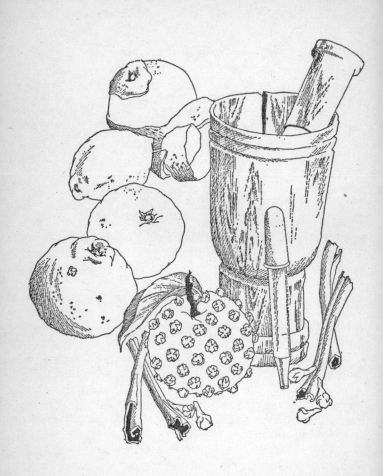

THE FRAGRANT CENTURIES

ONCE upon a time there were no supermarkets, no aerosol spray cans, no housing developments, no traffic jams, no launderettes; all the world worked hard and moved at horse-and-carriage pace. In the long still afternoons of summer, you heard crickets sing and the swish of wind in tall grasses. These were the centuries when candles lit the after-dark and the parlour was used only on Sunday.

In that far-off time, the mistress of the household was doctor and nurse and obstetrician as well as cook and mother. Pharmacist and perfumer, she made all the preparations that kept a home lovely and safeguarded her family's health – soaps and candles, medicines and mouth washes, moth repellents and disinfectants, cosmetics and powders and perfumes. With fragrant petals and herbs she scented her gloves and writing paper. Inks, linens and clothes were perfumed with sweet bags, and cakes and puddings and wines were flavoured with fragrant syrups. To 'make faire' musty rooms, she strewed rushes and sprinkled sweet-smelling vinegars and filled great bowls with rose petals and potpourris.

In Elizabethan homes, the fragrances were prepared in the 'stillroom'. It was a place where at least one small still could be kept, a warm room where flowers and herbs hung in bunches to dry, and long wooden shelves held row on row of mortars and pestles, fixatives, and exotic spices. Most of the information used in making the stillroom preparations the mistress of the household kept in her head. Some has come down to us in stillroom books where family knowledge of perfume and medicine, cooking and gardening was recorded from generation to generation.

In 1682 Mary Doggett wrote this 'receipt' for a 'sweet bagg' in one of the best known of the stillroom books. Exquisitely sophisticated, influenced by empires long gone even in Mary's day, it draws on knowledge men and women used to care for their homes and families very long ago.

Take half a pound of Cypress Roots, a pound of Orris, ¾ lb. Rhodium [rosewood], a lb. Coriander seed, ¾ lb. of Calamus, 3 oranges stuck with cloves [and probably dried on her still], 2 oz. of Benjamin, and an oz. of storax and 4 pecks of Damask Rose leaves, a peck of dryed sweet Marjerum, a pretty stick of Juniper shaved very thin, some lemon peel dryed; let all these be powdered very grosely for the first year and immediately put into your baggs; the next year pound and work it and it will be very good again.

Mary Doggett: Her Book of Recipes, 1682

The cinnamon-scented calamus Mary used in the 1600s is the ground root of the sweet flag, *Acorus calamus*, and it was one of the ingredients used by the children of Israel to make a holy anointing oil. In the Book of Exodus (30 : 23–4), as Moses led them across the great desert to the promised land, directions for making the perfume were recorded:

> Take thou also unto thee principal
> spices, of pure myrrh five hundred shekels,
> and of sweet cinnamon, half so much, . . .
> and of sweet calamus, two hundred and fifty
> and of cassia five hundred shekels, . . .
> and of olive oil, an hin [about one gallon].

In verse 34, there's another fragrant recipe that includes the 'sweet spices stacte and onycha and galbanum . . . with pure frankincense'.

These 'spices', which we think of as perfumes, were among the most precious possessions in biblical times. Myrrh, frankincense and gold were the three gifts the Wise Men of the East brought to the infant Jesus. As incense and holy oils, fragrances were used to invoke the protection of the gods and to drive away the evil spirits of illness and death.

Though this use of fragrance seems mystical, it had practical effects. The mistress of the Elizabethan stillroom would have completely understood this since she, too, battled sickness and plagues: the strongly scented fumes of burnt offerings and holy oils used in the ancient world to fumigate the temples and holy places where crowds gathered would have had some value in keeping sickness from spreading. The nomadic Hebrew and the Elizabethan both knew that where strong, good scents are, illness and insects frequently are not.

The desert dweller of biblical times used this information in ingenious ways and developed many of the scents that appeared centuries later in the stillrooms of England.

Bathing in the desert without water was achieved by squatting with garments tented over a hole in the sand where aromatics smouldered: the rising fumes caused a mighty perspiration that cleansed the skin, and the strong scent fumigated the body and clothing. To keep bedding and garments sweet-smelling and free of insects, the desert dwellers placed bags of aromatics in folds in the fabrics – a practice Homer reported in the *Odyssey*. (There's a fine Puritanical line drawn in the Bible between what makes for cleanliness and what makes for sin: The Book of Proverbs warns against the lures of the woman who perfumes her bed with myrrh and cinnamon and aloes.)

The fragrances that the Hebrews used – and probably had acquired during their Egyptian captivity – were primarily balsam and cinnamon that came from fragrant resins and barks. The aloe, a desert plant with spikes of flowers and a bitter juice, yields a balsam fragrance, as does *Boswellia*, the source of frankincense. Galbanum made from *Galbanum officinale* or from the milky fluid of a perennial, *Ferula galbaniflua*, is balsam-scented, too. Cassia oil, from *Cinnamomum cassia*, has a cinnamon fragrance, like Mary Doggett's calamus. The 'spice' called 'cinnamon' is probably one derived from the bark of an evergreen, *Cinnamomum glanduliferum*. Stacte (droppings) was an unguent made of myrrh and *origanum*, oregano; and onycha came from a small mollusc found on the shores of the Red Sea. Myrrh, an aromatic scent when warmed, is a resinous gum exuded by *Commonophora*.

The most treasured of these biblical perfumes was spikenard, the oil with which Mary Magdalene anointed the head of the Nazarene as he sat at dinner at the home of Simon the Leper. It was a scent somewhere between patchouli and valerian. All the way from the Himalayas, it was surely the most valuable possession the courtesan owned. Almost as expensive was labdanum, a balsam scent that was once the most common base for eastern perfumes. It is a sticky substance exuded by the rock-rose, *Cistus ladaniferus*. In biblical times, and in the Elizabethan and Victorian ages as well, it was gathered from goats allowed to graze among the plants where they collected it on their hairy coats and beards.

These ancient spices and perfumes survived the centuries from Moses to Elizabeth I and appeared in another housewife's recipe book, *The Toilet of Flora*, published in 1775. Flora left us not only a recipe, but a complete record of the plants that were used to fill 'little bags or satchels'. Made of muslin and tied to the backs of chairs or placed in drawers, the little bags helped perfume Flora's airless dining room and kept her bed-chamber and linens sweet.

Flora's Ingredients for Little Bags or Satchels

For this purpose may be used different parts of the Aromatic Plants; as Leaves of Southernwood, Dragon-wort, Balm, Mint, both garden and wild, Dittany, Ground-Ivy, Bay, Hyssop, Lovage, Sweet Marjoram, Origanum, Pennyroyal, Thyme, Rosemary, Savory, Scordium, and Wild Thyme. The Flowers of the Orange, Lemon, Lime and Citron Tree, Saffron, Lavender, Roses, Lily of the Valley, Clove-july flower, Wall-flower, Jonquil, and Mace. Fruits, as Aniseeds, etc. The Rings of Lemons, Oranges, etc. Small green Oranges, Juniper-berries, Nutmegs, and Cloves, Roots of Acorus, Bohemian Angelice, Oriental Costus, Sweet Flag, Orrice, Zedoary, etc. The Woods of Rhodium, Juniper, Cassia, St. Lucia, Sanders, etc. Gums, as Frankincense, Myrrh, Storax, Benjamin, Labdanum, Ambergrise, and Amber. Barks, as Canella Alba, Cinnamon, etc. Care must be taken that all these ingredients are perfectly dry, and kept in a dry place. To prevent their turning black, add a little common Salt. When you choose to have any particular flower predominant, a greater quantity of that plant must be used in proportion to the other ingredients.

Flora and her friends had some exotic ingredients and a surprising amount of information at their fingertips. They knew where to find and how to use scented wild grasses and herbs such as mint and balm and thyme. They could get oranges, lemons, and limes, which originated in warmer climates than theirs. In addition to the biblical perfumes, they used storax and benjamin, which, with a knowledge of the medicinal herbs, were a heritage from ancient Greece. (In old recipes, storax sometimes means gum benzoin [p. 31], sometimes *Styrax officinalis*, a vanilla-like scent, and sometimes *Levant storax*, a balsam, or piney scent.) The stillroom lady was neither isolated nor ignorant; she was a versatile and immensely knowledgeable person.

Our word 'perfume' is from the Latin, 'through smoke', and it was probably as smoke that fragrance was first appreciated. The Egyptians and Greeks scented their burnt offerings to the gods, even before the Romans. In view of such antiquity, it is not surprising that a wealth of myths and legends is associated with fragrant plants and perfumes. Circe, the enchantress, employed perfume to keep Odysseus from his travels, and, according to Greek legend, Helen of Troy acquired her fatal beauty from a perfume recipe given to her by Venus, the goddess of Love. Both men and women used scents, even the tough young conqueror Alexander the Great. Alexander had the floor of his quarters sprinkled with sweet water, an Eastern custom the Elizabethans adopted more than 1,500 years later, and Alexander's clothes were fumigated and scented with the smoke of myrrh and other fragrant resins. One recipe for perfume left to us from ancient Greece is for a scent favoured by men. Recorded in Pliny's *Natural History*, it was made of red-flowered lilies, oil of ben (*Styrax benzoin*), myrrh, and essences of roses, cinnamon, and saffron, from the saffron crocus.

The Greeks loved flowers and used them lavishly for fragrance, as did the Elizabethans in later centuries. At banquets, rose petals rained from the ceiling, guests wore crowns of flowers, and wines were scented with fresh violets, grown commercially to fill these many needs. Little muslin bags – like Flora's scented satchels – were set by every guest, and perfumes were passed to each. The Greek matron, like her stillroom sister, kept clothes in coffers made of fragrant wood, and perfumed clothing and bedclothes with the powdered root of the Florentine iris.

The Greek knowledge of perfume came from contact with Egypt and reached Europe by way of the Romans. The important contribution the Greeks made to stillrooms was the herbal lore that they collected and catalogued.

Egyptians were the most lavish users of perfume in all antiquity. They absorbed massive quantities of fragrant ingredients and salves in their elaborate burial rituals and for cosmetics. In the Imperial palaces along the Nile, guests were crowned with the exquisitely scented Sacred Blue Lotus and halls were made fragrant with potpourris of roses and aromatics. Cleopatra, who used perfume to seduce Caesar and later Mark Antony, carried the rose-bowl concept to extremes. To welcome Antony, she had the floors of her apartments strewn knee-deep in rose petals. For state occasions the seductive queen followed the Egyptian custom and had the purple sails of her barge washed in scented water. But we have little record of the way the Egyptians used the herbs on which the stillroom mistress depended.

In the rocky soil and strong sunshine of Greece, herbs grew well. The Greek living room opened onto a garden of fragrant herbs, for the Greeks also believed that where there were sharp, clean scents people stayed healthy. There is an Athenian tradition that the city was once saved from plague by the burning of herbs.

Fenugreek, which we use to flavour foods, was made into unguents by the Greeks, and extracts and essences of marjoram and mint, thyme and rosemary (an ingredient in modern colognes), were used as personal scents.

The Romans, conquering Greece, adopted the floral fragrances and enjoyed all the sybaritic uses that the Egyptians and Greeks had made of perfume. At the height of Roman power, Egypt shipped roses by the boatload across the Mediterranean to supply banquet halls where rose petals filled the air and fountains splashed perfume instead of water. Many of the ways of the Roman matron with herbs and fragrance drifted down the centuries to the stillroom, and are preserved in herbals. She scented clothes and bedding, with orris powder as a perfume and fixative; she made perfumed candles and burned aromatics in her home. The bay leaf with which she crowned Roman victors kept the plague 'at bay' and also made a soothing bath. Bay was used by the Elizabethans as a strewing herb to keep away sickness. And it was the Romans who gave the clove-scented pink to the Elizabethans – and posterity; dianthus was discovered during a Roman campaign near the Bay of Biscay in Spain and brought home to flavour Roman wines. In the Middle Ages, the pretty little pink was the 'sops' served by English taverns in 'sops in wine'. In early recipes it is one of the clove-scented flowers called 'gillyflower' from the French word for clove tree, *giroflier*.

The earliest complete herbal – a record of the uses of herbs – was written in the first century after Christ by a Greek, Dioscorides. Another compiled before the sixth century is signed Pseudo-Apuleius. It was translated into Anglo-Saxon in the eleventh century and many manuscripts and printed editions were available to the ladies of the stillrooms in the twelfth and thirteenth centuries. In the years just before Elizabeth I came to the throne two English herbals appeared, *The Grete Herbal* in 1526, and *Banckes's Herbal* in 1525. Browsing through these old health and welfare manuals, you catch a glimpse of the world the stillroom ladies dealt with – a world where poor sanitation and the spoilage of foods were fought along with such modern ills as insomnia, depression, and falling hair.

For fevers, *Banckes's Herbal* recommends people to 'heat oil of violet meddled with powder of poppy seeds'. Violets were prescribed for sore eyes, falling fits and drunkenness as well. Rosemary leaves put 'under thy bed's head . . . shalt deliver thee of all evil dreams'. The leaves of the Madonna lily 'being applied do help the serpent bitten', and will 'cause the hair to grow in used-up places'. Lavender was recommended to protect clothes, 'from dirty, filthy beasts', and also 'it preserves chastity . . . if the head is sprinkled with lavender water.' Apoplexy and palsy and loss of speech would give way to its 'strange unspeakable virtue'.

For poisoning rats, monkshood (aconite) was used, and black hellebore was for 'killing wolves and foxes', as well as for 'ye Epileptical, Melancholicall, Frantic, Arthritical, Paralyticall', and for curing gout, 'scruff of the head', and scabies. Aloes juice, when you could get it, was a help in 'procuring sleep', and preventing 'the hair from falling off', and 'worms in the belly and ears'. It was believed effective, too, for 'ill colour caused of the coldness of the stomach'.

Lice were a severe problem, and larkspur was widely used to combat them. (A concoction of stavesacre, or larkspur, seed is still a recognized remedy for head lice.) The wallflower, *Cheiranthus cheiri*, one of the clove-scented plants called gillyflower, was considered excellent medicine, particularly the lemon-coloured varieties. 'The juice of the flowers put in the eyes takes away the wicked specks therein,' and the water of the flowers 'drunk noon and night for three or four weeks doth cause women to be fruitful'. It was recommended to the Elizabethans to mitigate the hard labour of childbirth and also for paralysis, dropsy, and 'the chaps which are in the seat'.

Vervain, the herbals promised, 'for him that useth it, it will make a good breath', and it also would give to they who carried it 'love and grace of good mastres'. The root and leaves put into wine and the wine sprinkled about the house where the 'eating is' would make 'all merry'.

The stillroom lady kept close to nature, her traditional ally in the battle for her family's health and happiness. From the fields in the long hot days of summer she gathered rushes and sweet-smelling grasses to strew on her floors. In her gardens she grew medicinal herbs and flowers and aromatic plants with a thousand uses. In the fragrant stillroom she powdered, and mixed, and distilled; in winter, sitting by the fire, she put together from her summer harvests tussie-mussies and moth bags.

We've inherited dozens of lovely ways with dry perfumes and petals from the stillroom lady and her sister of later, less embattled centuries. They stitched sachets and edged them with lace, filled sweet bags with southernwood and lavender for linens, sewed scents into muslin envelopes to perfume leather and books and writing papers, made herb pillows and herb baths and herb vinegars against sickness, brewed herbal teas of lemon balm and alfalfa and mint. They simmered sweet-smelling candles and, to fill the rooms with the fragrance of flowers and fresh air, they made hundreds of potpourris and sweet jars.

We can buy modern variations of most of the stillroom products. Yet the things we make with our hands are often the things we value most. Our lives are richer when somewhere in our mechanized, commercial, antiseptic and unbelievably efficient lives, we can make space for the Elizabethan's quiet little corner of summer and sunshine – a stillroom for the making of potpourris and the compounding of sweet scents from the garden.

2
The Potpourris

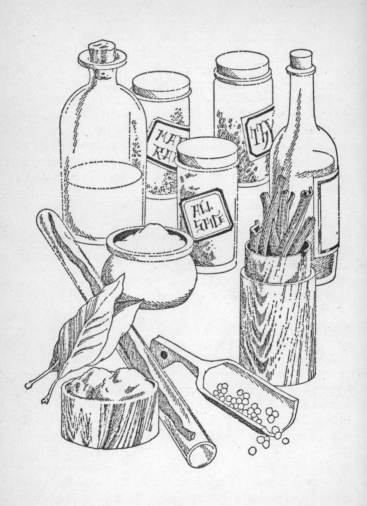

THE POTPOURRIS

A POTPOURRI – the French word is pronounced 'po poo ree' – has a quiet fragrance. You walk into a room and you may not know it is there, but after a while you say, 'What is that lovely scent?'

The potpourri, the sweet jar (or pot), and the rose bowl are referred to as potpourris. They are all made of fragrant dried petals. Potpourris and sweet jars are mixtures of several kinds of flowers and fragrant ingredients. The rose bowl includes mainly rose petals, or rose petals plus another ingredient or two, often lavender.

Potpourri recipes nearly always begin with rose petals. Roses most readily keep their fragrance when dried, while other richly perfumed flowers do not. At least, that was true of roses in the stillroom days when they, along with Madonna lilies and the few other flowers then grown, were classed as 'herbs' and only truly fragrant species were planted. Today there are not so many truly fragrant flowers, and the scent in most potpourris comes from fragrant oils.

The early Egyptian potpourri was made with rose petals and aromatics such as myrrh and the biblical fragrances. Ancient Greece and Rome added fixatives such as orris-root powder, storax, and benzoin, which held or fixed the volatile oils of fragrant materials so that they remained in the potpourri for years. The ladies of the stillroom were accustomed to scenting their homes with sweet bags and bowls filled with fragrant herbs, and they added herbs to their rose-petal mixtures. In the early 1500s after the Portuguese Vasco Da Gama had sailed around the coast of Africa and re-opened the spice trade with the East, spices appeared in potpourris, and in time the strongly scented animal fixatives – musk from the musk deer, ambergris from the sperm whale, civet from the civet cat –

came into use. However, not all potpourris use all these types of ingredients, and not all are made the same way. There are two basic methods for making potpourris: a moist method and a dry method.

The moist-method potpourri is the true potpourri, for the word *potpourri* means, literally, 'rotted pot'. *Pot* is a pot or a jar, and *pourri* is translated 'rotted' or 'fermented'. The moist method is more trouble and produces a less visually attractive potpourri, but, to my mind, the results offer a more subtle fragrance, and a fragrance that lasts longer.

There are any number of variations on the moist potpourri, but here is the basic procedure:

MOIST METHOD

Step 1. Pick and dry rose petals to a leathery texture: this takes about two days if the weather is dry. The petals will reduce in bulk by about 50 per cent.

Step 2. Layer the half-dried rose petals with salt (p. 35) in a large crock using about 1 scant cup of salt to 3 packed cupfuls of petals. Fill the crock about two thirds full.

Step 3. Store the crock in a dry, dark place for 10 days. It should be well ventilated to avoid the danger of mildew. The petals will usually cake and they are the base for your potpourri.

Step 4. Break up the caked base. Add to it the other ingredients, the spices and fixatives. Seal and store for 6 weeks, frequently shaking or mixing. This is the curing process.

Step 5. Next, add essential oils and other dried flowers, unless, as in some recipes, you've been instructed to add them in *Step 4*. Seal and cure another 2 weeks.

The potpourri is now ready to be transferred to decorative containers. Keep close covered at all times, except when opened for use.

Dry potpourris and rose bowls are made with absolutely bone dry petals. There are many variations of the dry method, too. This is the basic procedure:

DRY METHOD

Step 1. Pick and dry the petals until they are as crackly as corn-flakes. It will take about 10 days depending on the thickness of the petals and the dryness of the weather. They will reduce in bulk by 60 per cent, or more.

Step 2. Combine the petals with all other ingredients – spices, herbs, fixatives, fragrant oils – and mix well.

Step 3. Seal into a crock or a plastic bag, and store for 6 weeks, daily shaking gently. The potpourri is now ready for transfer to decorative containers. Keep close covered at all times, except when opened for use.

Following either the moist or the dry method, you can develop your own potpourri recipes with any fragrant flowers from your garden. The only additional information you need is the role the ingredients play in the composition of potpourri.

BASIC POTPOURRI INGREDIENTS

FLOWERS, HERBS AND SPICES

These are added by cupful or spoonful (p. 11) and are the body of the potpourri. The most plentiful ingredient governs the bouquet or fragrance of the potpourri. It can be rose or a combination of rose and lavender, or a mixture of several other flowers and herbs.

Most potpourris include roses and lavender because these best retain their fragrance when dried. Rosebuds, which dry into exquisite miniatures in delicate shadings of pink and green, have no scent and are only included for colour and texture. (I buy them if possible, rather than sacrifice so many unopened roses from my garden.) The petals of clove pinks, *Dianthus caryophyllus*, jasmine and orange blossoms are excellent. (See Chapter 7, Table C, for a list of other fragrant flowers.)

The herbs add body and their own particular qualities to the bouquet. Most often used are lemon verbena and rose geranium, rosemary and sweet marjoram, peppermint, bay, lemon balm, lemon geranium, lemon thyme, sweet basil, sweet woodruff, and tarragon.

The third element in the bouquet is the scent of spices. Most often used are cloves, cinnamon, allspice, nutmeg. When several of them are added, they are generally called for in equal amounts. A common proportion is 1 tablespoonful of spices to 4 cupfuls of flower petals and herbs. Cardamom, coriander and anise are sometimes part of oriental mixtures.

With just a few of these basic ingredients – petals, herbs, spices – and nothing else, you can make a lovely potpourri as long as your flower petals are from really fragrant varieties. The perfumes are faint, subtle, and charming. A favourite of Catherine of Braganza, Charles II's wife, was made with three parts 'of a basin' of rose petals dried in an airy room away from strong sunlight, to which were added a cupful of dried rosemary, of thyme, and of lavender, together with the dried and powdered skin of an orange and some cloves.

Orange rind, and lemon or lime as well, add a faint fragrance, and are called for in many early recipes. A nineteenth-century recipe that would be fun to try, if one had fresh orange blossoms handy, uses only cloves, the rind of a lemon, and fragrant flowers and herbs. It is made by the moist method.

Sweet Pot

Take three handsful of orange-flowers, three of clove-gilly flowers [clove pinks], three of damask roses, one of knotted marjoram, one of myrtle [sweet myrtle], half one of mint, one of lavender, the rind of a lemon, and a quarter of an ounce of cloves. Chop all and put them in layers, with pounded bay-salt between, up to the top of the jar. If all the ingredients cannot be got at once, put them in as you get them; always throwing in salt with every new article.

Domestic Cookery, 1834

FIXATIVES

The oils that carry fragrance are volatile and rapidly disappear without the presence of an agent that absorbs and holds them, a 'fixative'. Most fixatives have a scent of their own that becomes part of the 'bouquet' of the potpourri – so the amount of any one fixative used depends on how many other fixatives are called for.

In earlier centuries three popular fixatives were musk, civet, and ambergris, but they are not favoured today. You will probably find it difficult to obtain tinctures of these fixatives nowadays, though Caswell-Massey, an old-established American firm of chemists and perfumers, lists them in its mail-order catalogue (p. 125). (Vegetable oils which simulate them are, however, quite widely available.) On its own, each has an unpleasant odour, but in a potpourri they introduce a rich, illusive scent. Many interesting old recipes call for one or another of them. They are added by the drop, and just one drop too many can ruin a whole potpourri.

More popular today are the vegetable fixatives. Orris-root powder is the most common. You should be able to buy supplies of this (and of gum benzoin which is described below) from the sources listed on p. 125, but you can also make it yourself if you grow the blue-flowered *Iris florentina*, a variety of the familiar *Iris germanica*. Dig up the roots, peel them carefully, and dry them in the sun. Store them in a dry airy place for a year or two; the fragrance is stronger the second year. Then grind or powder the root as needed. About a third of a cup is used for 4 to 8 cups of petals.

Gum benzoin is another popular fixative and is often used along with orris-root. Early recipes call it 'benjamin', and some recipes call for 'oil of ben'. A resin from the benzoin tree, *Styrax benzoin*, native to the Far East, it is sold as gum benzoin today (p. 125 for suppliers). It has an aromatic scent. About 30 grammes (1 ounce) to 8 or 12 cups of petals is a common proportion.

The tonka bean, or tonquin bean, from *Dipterix odorata*, is another modern fixative. The extract once flavoured snuffs and tobaccos; the scent is variously described as resembling that of flowers or of vanilla. In any case, it is aromatic and sweet. One or two beans are all that most recipes call for.

Other ingredients that are classed as fragrances, but act as fixatives and are used as such, include the old biblical 'spices' frankincense and myrrh, sandalwood, patchouli, oakmoss and vetiver. They are described below.

Frankincense, today called olibanum, is the main ingredient in religious incense. Like myrrh – which gives fragrance only when warm – it is sold by G. Baldwin and Co. (p. 125). Frankincense and myrrh appear rarely in modern recipes, but Elizabethan recipes often include them.

Sandalwood, from *Santalum album*, a small parasitic tree found in India, is called 'santal' in some recipes. The scent is easy to detect, once you know it, but hard to describe. We think of it as 'oriental'. Culpeper sell sandalwood raspings (p. 125); you may also find it for sale in powdered form. For dry earthy potpourris, between 25 and 50 grammes – about an ounce or two – is what most recipes call for.

Patchouli leaves, from the shrubby *Pogostemon cablin*, have a musky, woodsy smell that combines well with roses and is lovely in small doses. A few leaves are as much as any potpourri can take. About 25 to 50 grammes (an ounce or two) is called for with 8 to 16 cups of petals. If leaves, powder or shavings are not available, substitute an essence.

Oakmoss, a fixative known as chypre or cypre, is a fragrant moss called *Evernia pranastri*, used in perfume-making. You may well find it difficult to obtain supplies. I cannot recommend a specific substitute but tonka beans or broken cinnamon sticks might be nice used in its place. Again, 25 to 50 grammes (an ounce or two) is a usual quantity. Baldwin's (p. 125) stock an oakmoss fragrance.

Vetiver is a sweet-smelling grass, *Vetiveria zizanioides*, whose fragrant root has a scent like violets or sandalwood. It is normally used in shreds or raspings. Vetiver *can* be grown in the greenhouse, so you may like to try cultivating your own stock if by any chance you can get a root of it. About 25 to 50 grammes (an ounce or two) of vetiver is right for most pot-pourris. (Baldwin's stock a vetiver fragrance.)

Any fixative material left over from potpourri making can be used in the recipes for sachets and other fragrances given in Chapters 5 and 6.

ESSENTIAL OILS

Because many of the showy flowers in our gardens are less fragrant than species grown in earlier centuries, modern re-cipes generally call for essences of flowers and other scents. If you have highly fragrant petals, cut down on the amount of essential oil called for.

The terms 'oil of', 'essential oil of' and 'essence of' are often used loosely for the same thing: an oil with a very strong scent – so strong, it generally isn't pleasant used alone or in quantity. The strength and quality differ with each supplier; the price may do so too (generally because of a real difference in quality). For this reason I have been very conservative in the amounts of oil or essence called for in these recipes. Use essential oils sparingly – it is impossible to remove a drop of oil of roses from a bowlful of dried flowers if you've overdone it. Add the amount of oil called for a drop at a time, and smell the fragrance as you go. How much is too much depends on your own highly personal sense of smell – and also on the other ingredients in the potpourri. The addition of 6 drops of essence is enough for a lot of dried flowers – at least 8 cups. It is safer to start with 4 drops and then, if you wish, to add one drop more, even two, to suit your own taste.

A great many scents are available in the form of essences. There is a note about suppliers on p. 125. Essences of rose, lavender, patchouli, rose geranium, rosemary, sandalwood, musk, violet, cedarwood, lemon verbena and others are generally available; range, strength and quality will differ from supplier to supplier. You can often use an essence, in minute quantities, to replace dry ingredients that you may not be able to locate. For instance, musk oil can be used instead of grains of musk. An essence is a helpful substitute when you are working with old recipes whose ingredients are hard to find.

Suppliers (Baldwin's, for instance) may also stock a pot-pourri oil or essence of potpourri. Allow 5 drops of any such essence to 8 cups of any dried flowers available to make a quick – and lovely – potpourri. To turn the essence into a classical dry potpourri, add 2 cups of lemon verbena leaves, 1 cup of dried rosemary leaves, 1 tablespoon of dried and grated lemon peel, $\frac{1}{3}$ cup of orris-root powder, and 1 table-spoon each of crushed clove, nutmeg, ginger and cinnamon.

As a general rule, do not double the amount of any one essential oil even if you double the number of cupfuls of petals. Rather, add other fragrant fixatives or a few drops of another essence.

DRIED FLOWERS AND PETALS

Two cupfuls of dried flowers added purely for colour and texture improve the look of almost any potpourri. You add these to a moist potpourri when it is finished, and to a dry potpourri before curing. Table E at the back of the book lists flowers to dry for colour. Among the best and easiest to find in today's gardens are delphinium and larkspur, violets, pan-sies, dianthus, bachelor's buttons and blue mallow. I particu-larly like the deep colour of dried zinnia petals, and suggest marigolds as well because so many gardeners grow them. From mail-order suppliers (see p. 125) you can buy dried flowers, such as rosebuds, marigolds and elder blossoms. Alternatively you can dry your own, as described in Chapters 3 and 4.

HANDLING POTPOURRI INGREDIENTS

Drying petals. Picking and drying flowers for the moist method is detailed in Chapter 3; for the dry method, see Chapter 4.

Spices. Fresh whole spices, coarsely ground in a pepper mill or pounded in a mortar, are more fragrant than tired old powdered spices from supermarket shelves. Powdered spices generally cloud a crystal container; if the recipe calls for powdered ingredients, the potpourri will probably look best in an opaque container.

Citrus peel. Either pare this with a vegetable peeler, carefully discarding any white pith, or grate the coloured peel off the fruit. In ancient recipes the citrus was usually dried and crushed or minced. I coat pared peel with orris-root powder and either dry it in very low oven (100 to 120°F) or put it on racks in a dry, airy room and let time do the drying.

Salt. Potpourris need a very coarse salt that does not absorb too much moisture. Old recipes call for bay salt. In *Magic Gardens*, Rosetta E. Clarkson describes bay salt as the coarsest grade obtained in a process that runs water over salt rocks, then boils it down to brine. Other authorities consider bay salt synonymous with sea salt. I have used coarse kosher salt as a substitute (this is a very coarse, pure salt that seems not to hold too much moisture), mixed half and half with non-iodized fine table salt, for moist potpourris and when bay salt is called for. Coarse sea salt, mixed half and half with fine non-iodized salt, is a perfectly suitable substitute. Any salt *should* do, but a non-iodized salt would be best.

PROPORTIONS

These generalizations are for use when making up your own potpourris. In the recipes in the chapters that follow, there are many deviations from these proportions because the ingredients called for vary, and also because there are many ways to make a good potpourri. There is a note about measures on p. 11.

Salt: To make a moist potpourri, 1 scant cupful to 3 packed cupfuls of fresh petals.

Spices: 1 tablespoon to 4 cups dried petals.

Powdered fixatives: $\frac{1}{3}$ cup to 4 to 8 cups petals.

Essential oils: 4 to 6 drops to 6 to 8 cups petals.

EQUIVALENTS

In working with old recipes I translate the quantities thus:

> *petals:* 1 handful = 1 cupful
> *spices and powdered fixatives:* 1 oz. (30 g) = $\frac{1}{3}$ cup
> *dried herbs, small, as lavender:* 1 oz. (30 g) = $\frac{3}{4}$ cup
> *dried leaves, medium, as basil:* 1 oz. (30 g) = 1 cup
> *petals and flowers, small, as chamomile:* 1 oz. (30 g) = 1 cup
> *rosebuds and large petals:* 1 oz. (30 g) = 1 cup;
>   1 quart = 4 oz. (120 g) = 4 cups

In metric terms, 1 ounce weighs just under 30 grammes, and 1 pound is almost exactly 450 grammes. Since 1 drachm equals $\frac{1}{16}$ ounce (avoirdupois), in metric terms it is a scant 2 grammes: an apothecaries' drachm, however, equals $\frac{1}{8}$ ounce (3·5 grammes).

BUYING

When buying essential oils, 10 millilitres (between $\frac{1}{4}$ and $\frac{1}{2}$ fluid ounce) will provide scent for several recipes. About 120 grammes (4 ounces) of spices and fixatives, except possibly orris-root, is enough to start with. Since you will need lots of flowers and petals, the economical way is to grow them yourself, and growing your own ingredients is part of the pleasure of making potpourris.

CONTAINERS FOR POTPOURRIS

The original potpourri jar was developed in the 1700s. It became so popular and so elaborate that it was a great attraction in royal palaces and the homes of the wealthy; it has been described as the apex of the porcelain-maker's art in France and England during the eighteenth century. The jars were usually mounted on bases. Exquisitely decorated with exotic birds, jar, lid and base were often encrusted with porcelain reproductions of the flowers included in the fragrant contents.

Most of the early containers had a close-fitting outer lid and a perforated inner cover. The outer lid was removed when the potpourri was in use, and the fragrance wafted through the holes in the inner lid.

Modern potpourris accent colour and texture as well as fragrance, and can be displayed attractively in crystal and glass containers as well as in small porcelain jars. If the potpourri is made the moist way, and is less than beautiful, you can still display it in crystal or glass containers if you line the glass with dried and pressed pansies or other flat-faced flowers and fasten them with a glue which dries clear.

Any crystal or glass bowl is a suitable container as long as it has a close-fitting lid to keep the perfume from escaping when the potpourri isn't in use. There are also some very attractive clear plastic containers and low-priced pretty storage glass jars, some stacked, which are lovely for the display of three or four kinds of potpourri. Apothecary bottles, as long as they are wide-mouthed, are suitable potpourri containers: these are usually stoppered with broad cork tops which you can lacquer if you wish. That ubiquitous denizen of the modern kitchen, the instant coffee jar, makes another attractive potpourri holder if you lacquer the top in a colour that suits the potpourri – old rose, soft blue, pale green, even gold.

Small new or antique ginger jars from China are ideal for moist potpourris. In antique shops you can also find tobacco jars, tin tea caddies, attractive old cigar boxes, small flower bowls. Charming old sugar bowls with lids and even thimble baskets can be used; line these with polythene film, and make a fabric cover lined with stiff cardboard that will fit tightly inside.

TO REVITALIZE
A FADING POTPOURRI

A well-made potpourri is said to last up to fifty years. If the fragrance fades in time, it can be revitalized with a few drops of its principal floral essence. A little brandy or eau de cologne added just before using brings out the scent of a dying potpourri. Floris (p. 126) sell a Reviver Essence for fading potpourri and you may like to try this too.

In *Delights for Ladies*, published in 1594, Sir Hugh Platt gives his ideas for retaining the perfume of a potpourri: '. . . you should hang your pot in an open chimney or near a continual fire so that the petals will keep exceeding fair in colour and be most delicate in scent.' In Sir Hugh's day the potpourri's main enemy was the humidity of damp, unheated rooms, and his is still good advice for the owner of a waterside house.

SOME EARLY RECIPES

Because potpourri has to be governed by the contents of the maker's garden, history has left us more suggestions for making potpourris than exact recipes. Anecdotes weave their way through the stories of romantic figures of the past.

There are a few recipes that go back through the centuries; each makes its own distinct and subtle fragrant statement. Try one when you feel you have enough experience to know how to substitute successfully for the ingredients that are no longer easily available. There is a note about equivalent measurements on p. 36.

The first recipe is almost all fixative and essence of scent.

Since the ingredients are mainly dry, the salt is intended to bulk out the preparation. I would omit much of the salt and add more of dried flowers. Bay salt was coarse, so I would substitute coarse sea salt.

Take of orris-root, flag-root [calamus], bruised, each 4 oz.; yellow sandal-wood, 3 oz.; sweet cedar-wood, 1 oz.; patchouli leaves, 1 oz. The above should be coarsely powdered and well mixed. Then add bay-salt, 1 lb.; rose leaves, 3 oz.; essence of lemon, half a drachm; millifleurs [try a potpourri essence or a concentrated potpourri oil], 1 drachm; oil of lavender, 20 drops; musk, 10 grains [4 drops essence of musk, adding more, a drop at a time, if wished].

The Practical Housewife, 1860

This next old recipe is fairly easy to duplicate. The only instruction omitted is curing time; I'd allow about six weeks. A peck was 2 gallons, dry measure, so you would need a lot of roses – about 32 cupsful. Failing balm of Gilead, try a little musk oil or essence of musk, used sparingly.

Put into a large China jar the following ingredients in layers, with bay-salt [see above] strewn between the layers; 2 pecks damask roses, part in buds, part full bloom; violets, orange-flowers, and jasmine, a handful each; orris-root sliced, benjamin and storax, two ounces each; a quarter of an ounce of musk [try essence of musk, added a drop at a time]; a quarter of a pound of angelica-root sliced; two handfuls of lavender flowers; bay and laurel leaves, half a handful each; three Seville oranges, stuck as full of cloves as possible, dried in a cool oven, and pounded; half a handful of knotted majoram; and two handfuls of balm of Gilead, dried. Cover all quite close. When the pot is uncovered, the perfume is very fine.

Domestic Cookery, 1834

You would have to have highly scented petals for the following recipe to work. For cypress-powder, I would substitute cedar (use a liquid cedar fragrance if wood or shavings are not available), and for violet powder, orris-root with oil of violet.

Take a pound of fresh-gathered Orange Flowers, of common roses, lavender seeds and musk roses, each half a pound; of Sweet marjoram leaves, and clove-gilly flowers [pinks] picked, each a quarter of a pound; of thyme, three ounces; of Myrtle [sweet myrtle] leaves, and Melilot stalks stripped of their leaves, each two ounces; of rosemary leaves, and cloves, bruised, each an ounce; of bay leaves, half an ounce. Let these ingredients be mixed in a large pan covered with parchment, and be exposed to the heat of the sun during the whole summer; for the first month stirring them every other day with a stick, and taking them within doors in rainy weather. Towards the end of the season they will afford an excellent composition for a perfume; which may be rendered yet more fragrant, by adding a little scented Cypress-powder, mixed with coarse violet-powder.

The Toilet of Flora, 1775

Rondelitia Potpourri

This was a popular perfume in the sixteenth century.

8 cups dried lavender
120 g (4 oz.) orris-root
75 g (2¾ oz.) vanilla bean
60 g (2 oz.) cloves

15 g (½ oz.) allspice
60 g (2 oz.) dried bergamot
8 cups dried rose petals
15 g (½ oz.) cinnamon

Since all the ingredients described here are dried, follow the dry method for potpourri (p. 29). If you cannot get bergamot, take 120 grammes (4 ounces) of orange peel, stick the cloves through the peelings, dry, and pound to powder; alternatively, use 4 to 6 drops of essence of bergamot, more if you feel the need for a stronger scent. Vanilla pod can be used in place of vanilla bean.

3
Moist Potpourris and Sweet Jars

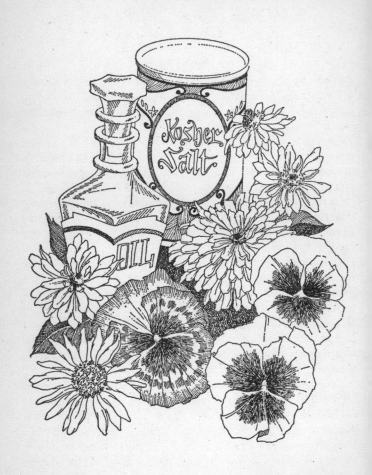

3

MOIST POTPOURRIS
AND SWEET JARS

PICK fresh, fragrant petals in the middle of the morning on a dry summer day, after the dew has evaporated and just before the garden begins to smell of roses, or else in the early evening before the dew falls.

One giant rose bush, well fed and in full sun, will produce enough roses in a season to make a good potpourri. The petals need not all go in at once; there are several recipes that allow you to gather the roses throughout a season.

In the past, only very fragrant roses were selected for potpourri. The Provence or cabbage rose, *Rosa centifolia*, was one of the best. It was known in colonial America, where it was called the hundred-leaved rose. (There was a gentleness in New England seafaring men that made them dig up roots and ask for seeds in every land they knew, so that their seaside home gardens bloomed with the pink Provence, and the red Provence, and also *damascena*, the damask rose, one of the most fragrant in the world.) Some moden hybrids of these and other highly fragrant species are listed in Table B of Chapter 7, and all are suitable for moist potpourris. Table C of Chapter 7 gives a list of other suitable fragrant flowers.

Fragrant petals for a moist potpourri are partially dried before they are measured. Herb leaves are usually completely dried (p. 57). (*All* ingredients for a dry potpourri are completely dried.) For drying, I use window screens; I lay the screens across the tops of chair backs in the attic. It is dark there, dry, warm, and well ventilated. Pull off the petals and spread them one deep across the screens. Cover them with cheesecloth raised on sundae glasses so the cloth does not actually touch the petals. If you have no window screens available, a good drying rack can be made by stretching cheese-cloth taut between two sawhorses; you can make a span as wide as the cloth, but don't make one so long that the weight of the petals sags the cloth and heaps the petals in the middle.

If the weather is dry, and the drying room warm and airy, the petals should be suitable for a moist potpourri in two days. They will have reduced in bulk by about half and will have a soft, leathery texture. They are now ready for the first step described in the moist recipes – layering with salt (p. 35). I use old ceramic jars for small mixtures. Beer crocks, which are straight-sided, are larger and good for making potpourris that consume a whole season's production of petals. When you are making a progressive potpourri – gathering, drying, and salt-layering petals as flowers come into bloom – stir up the previous batch before adding the new.

The salt-and-petal mixture will ferment and sometimes froth. If it froths, stir it well daily until the frothing stops, then allow the mixture to cure another 10 days. Eventually a cake or a caked mass will form. Take this out and crumble it before mixing in the remaining ingredients.

The petals don't always froth; sometimes they yield their moisture and dry out. The important thing is that the mass be dry – caked or layered in petal flakes – before the rest of the ingredients are added, *unless the recipe specifies otherwise*: in some recipes, the fragrant spices and fixatives *are* added earlier in the potpourri.

The recipes that follow offer a spectrum of the many, many ways in which moist potpourris have been made through the ages. Recipes with many fragrant oils and additives are apt to be rather expensive. They all have exquisite scents and make charming and very welcome gifts.

Potpourri with Brandy

A good season-long project for the gardener with a quantity of roses. This is a 1928 recipe and calls for brandy, which is supposed to bring up the fragrance. The sugar, an ingredient in many old recipes, is meant to assist the drying process and sweeten the scent.

32 cups fragrant rose petals
2 cups coarse salt
2 cups fine salt
4 tablespoons allspice
4 tablespoons ground cloves
4 tablespoons light brown sugar

⅔ cup orris-root powder
4 cups dried fragrant petals: lavender, lemon verbena, or orange blossoms
120 g (4 oz.) gum benzoin
55 ml (2 fl. oz.) fine brandy

As they are available, dry rose petals to a leathery texture. Mix coarse and fine salt. Layer petals as they dry in a big crock – about 7 litres (6 quarts). Cover each 12-millimetre (half-inch) layer with a sprinkling of salt. Keep the crock in a warm, dry, airy place, and stir the petals daily. When you have all the petals called for, all salted and dried, mix spices, sugar and orris-root powder and toss gently with the rose petals. Mix in the 4 cups of dried (bone dry) petals, then the gum benzoin. Seal and cure for 6 weeks. Toss with the brandy, and keep covered except when in use.

Rose Potpourri

This is an adaptation of a recipe from *Floral Magazine*, 1925, a standard rose potpourri. If your petals are not highly fragrant, add 3 or 4 drops of oil of roses when the potpourri is completed, and cure it for another two weeks.

6 cups fragrant rose petals
½ cup coarse salt
½ cup table salt
1 teaspoon ground cinnamon
½ teaspoon ground cloves

6 leaves dried lemon verbena
¼ cup dried rosemary
½ cup dried lavender
2 tablespoons orris-root powder
1 cup dried rosebuds

45

Dry the rose petals to a leathery texture. Combine coarse and fine salt. In a 2½-litre (4-pint) wide-mouthed crock, layer the petals with the salt. The petal layers should be about 12 millimetres (half an inch) deep. Set away in a dry, airy place for 10 days. Stir or shake daily. When the mixture is dry, crumble it and add the remaining ingredients. Seal and cure for 6 weeks. Transfer to a decorative container and keep covered except when in use.

Rose-and-Spice Potpourri

If your petals are very fragrant, you may not need 5 drops of rose oil.

8 cups rose petals	2 tablespoons ground cloves
¾ cup kosher salt or coarse sea salt	2 tablespoons ground nutmeg
	2 tablespoons ground allspice
¾ cup table salt	1 stick cinnamon, crushed
2 tablespoons ground mace	1 cup dried rosebuds
⅔ cup orris-root powder	5 drops rose oil

Dry the petals to a leathery texture. Combine coarse and fine salt. In a 3½-litre (6-pint) wide-mouthed crock, layer the petals with the salt, each layer about 12 millimetres (half an inch) deep. Set in a dry, airy place for 10 days, stirring daily. When the mixture is dry, crumble it and add remaining ingredients. Add the rose oil a drop at a time and mix well. Cure, sealed, for 6 weeks. Transfer to a decorative container and keep covered except when in use.

Rose Potpourri with Ginger

Ginger was a popular ingredient in many old fragrance recipes; it introduces a spicy, exotic scent. If your flowers are not very fragrant, add up to 6 drops of rose oil before the curing process.

12 cups red Provence rose petals	2 tablespoons ground clove
1 cup coarse salt	⅓ cup finely sliced fresh
1 cup fine salt	ginger root or ¼ cup
2 tablespoons ground	powdered ginger
cinnamon	4 tablespoons anise seed
2 tablespoons ground nutmeg	⅔ cup powdered orris-root

Dry the rose petals to a leathery texture. Mix coarse and fine salt. Layer petals about 12 millimetres (half an inch) deep, with a sprinkling of salt over each layer. Store in a dry, dark, airy place for 10 days, or until petals have dried. Stir daily while drying. Mix in the remaining ingredients. Seal the jar and cure for 6 weeks before using. Keep covered when not in use.

Rose Potpourri with Cologne

The procedure here is different: a drying mixture is prepared and the fresh, undried petals are added as available. The fragrance is rather heavy.

Grated rind of 2 lemons	10 g (⅓ oz.) dried lavender
1 cup coarse salt	55 ml (2 fl. oz.)
1 cup fine salt	lavender cologne
⅓ cup powdered orris-root	55 ml (2 fl. oz.)
30 g (1 oz.) gum benzoin	eau de cologne
¼ cup ground cinnamon	14 ml (½ fl. oz.) bergamot oil
¼ cup ground cloves	8 drops tincture of musk or
¼ cup ground nutmeg	oil of musk
12 bay leaves	2 cups rosebuds, dried
¼ teaspoon dried sage	12 cups fresh fragrant
¼ teaspoon dried rosemary	rose petals
¼ teaspoon dried mint	

Mix everything thoroughly except the rose petals. Seal into a 3½-litre (6-pint) crock; keep in a warm, airy room. As you acquire your petals, stir them gently into the mixture. Keep only lightly covered, so a little air can get to the petals; stir daily with a wooden spoon. (But I'm not sure a wooden spoon is essential!) When all the roses have been added and are fairly well dried, cover the jar and cure for 2 to 3 months before using.

A Very Fragrant Potpourri

This one is highly fragrant and also quite expensive because of the cost of the essential oils. Allspice (the berry of *Pimenta officinalis*) is pounded in a mortar just enough to crack open the berries. If you cannot get grains of musk and tincture of musk, use a musk oil or essence of musk instead – about 3 to 4 drops, added carefully, a drop at a time; check the fragrance as you go. If you cannot get oil of bergamot, try the substitute described on p. 40. Just a little of this potpourri scents a room. It will easily take another 4 cups of dried petals, any kind, if you want to stretch it. Add them when the curing process is over.

16 *cups fragrant rose petals*
6 *cups any highly scented flowers*
3 *cups coarse salt*
3 *cups fine salt*
1 *cup broken allspice*
⅔ *cup coarse-ground cinnamon*
½ *cup coarse-ground nutmeg*
½ *cup whole cloves*
⅓ *cup anise seeds*
10 *grains musk*
6 *cups dried lavender*
⅔ *cup orris-root powder*

8 *patchouli leaves* or 2 *drops patchouli oil*
14 *ml* (½ *fl. oz.*) *oil of bergamot*
7 *ml* (¼ *fl. oz.*) *oil of rose geranium* or ¼ *cup dried rose geranium leaves*
7 *ml* (¼ *fl. oz.*) *oil of lavender*
7 *ml* (¼ *fl. oz.*) *oil of lemon*
3.5 *ml* (⅛ *fl. oz.*) *tincture of musk*
7 *ml* (¼ *fl. oz.*) *oil of rosemary*
8 *drops oil of roses*

Dry the rose petals to a leathery texture. Mix coarse and fine salt. Layer petals, 12 millimetres (half an inch) deep, in a 7-litre (12-pint) crock, sprinkling each with salt. Set in a dark, dry, airy place. Stir twice daily. After 7 days, mix in allspice and the cinnamon. Cover the crock and cure for a week, tossing lightly daily. Add all the other ingredients, including the oils. Mix well. Seal, and cure for 6 weeks more before using. Keep potpourri covered unless in use.

Potpourri with a Dry Fragrance

Much less flowery than most mixtures, this is a recipe that begins with the preparation of a drying mixture, to which petals are then added. Fragrant oils make it rather expensive – and quite heady. If you cannot get bergamot oil, try the substitute described on p. 40.

⅓ cup ground allspice
⅓ cup ground nutmeg
1¼ cups orris-root powder
Grated rind of 3 lemons
14 ml (½ fl. oz.) oil of
   rose geranium or 1 cup
   dried rose geranium leaves

½ cup coarse salt
½ cup fine salt
14 ml (½ fl. oz.) lemon oil
14 ml (½ fl. oz.) bergamot oil
14 ml (½ fl. oz.) lavender oil
32 cups petals of roses or other
   flowers

Mix everything but the rose petals in a large crock – about 14 litres (3 gallons); keep it sealed in a warm, dry, dark place. As petals become available, stir them into the mixture, tossing well. Keep the jar covered, but not sealed, and stir daily. When all the petals have been added, cover lightly and stir daily until the mixture seems quite dry. Then cover and cure for 8 weeks before using. Keep covered when not in use.

Potpourri for a Big Garden

This is a recipe for the gardener with many flowers to spare; it is intended to be made over the entire season of bloom. Substitute additional rose petals or petals from clove pinks for any of these you don't have. Use any lemon-scented leaf, like lemon verbena, if you don't have a lemon tree handy to supply leaves. Rose water is available from a chemist's.

2 cups narcissus
2 cups jonquils
2 cups lily of the valley
2 cups fragrant blue lilac
2 cups fragrant white lilac
2 cups orange blossoms
2 cups mignonette
2 cups heliotrope
2 cups balm leaves (Melissa officinalis)
2 cups clove pinks
2 cups acacia flowers
2 cups lemon leaves

2 cups red rose petals
2 cups pink rose petals
2 cups moss rose petals
2 cups damask rose petals
1 cup rosemary
1 cup thyme
1 cup sweet myrtle leaves
2½ cups coarse salt
2½ cups fine salt
2½ cups orris-root powder
3 cups rose water, or *6 drops rose oil*

Pick the flowers as they come into bloom and dry to a leathery texture. Mix coarse and fine salt and orris-root powder. Layer the flowers, each layer about 12 millimetres (half an inch) deep, in a 14-litre (3-gallon) crock, sprinkling each layer with salt–orris-root mixture. Allow about 1 cup of this mixture to each 2½ cups of flowers. Stir daily through the season, and store in a dark, dry, airy place. When the pot-pourri is complete, and has dried out, moisten with rose water, or add rose oil, stirring it in well. Then seal the jar and cure for 2 weeks before using. Keep covered when not in use.

Potpourri Made with Borax

Borax is a drying agent for preserving flowers, and that is its purpose here. In this recipe, the salt and borax are mixed, and petals and herbs added as available.

2 cups coarse salt
2 cups borax
⅓ cup coarse-ground cinnamon
¼ cup dried rose geranium leaves
½ cup dried lemon verbena
    leaves

½ cup dried thyme
½ cup dried bay leaves, broken
1 cup dried lavender flowers
6 drops rose oil
12 cups fragrant rose petals
1 cup dried rosebuds

Mix the salt and borax and cinnamon in a 5-litre (1-gallon) crock. Seal and keep in a warm, dry place. In a separate crock place the fragrant leaves and lavender flowers, all chopped fine. Add the rose oil. Seal and store. As rose petals become available, mix into the salt, borax, and cinnamon mixture. Stir daily as petals dry. When all the rose petals have been added, stir in the dried herb mixture and add the rosebuds. Seal and cure for 6 weeks. Keep covered when not in use.

European Rose Jar

Most chemists sell glycerine, the kind for chapped hands and lips. If damask rose petals are not available, add 6 drops of rose oil before curing. Grain alcohol, also known as ethyl alcohol and as ethanol, is expensive and may prove difficult to obtain. A good chemist *should* be able to order it for you; failing this, try the local chemical suppliers to see if any of them will sell small quantities to the general public or can advise on possible sources of supply.

6 drops oil of rose geranium
    or ½ cup dried rose
    geranium leaves
6 drops of glycerine
32 cups fresh damask rose
    petals
1½ cups grain alcohol
3 cups coarse salt
¼ cup broken allspice (see p. 48)

¼ cup coarse-ground nutmeg
¼ cup coarse-ground
    cinnamon
¼ cup orris-root powder
1 cup dried lavender flowers
¼ cup dried heliotrope
4 cups dried rosebuds
2 cups dried lemon verbena
    leaves

Select a decorative bowl that will hold about 11 litres (2½ gallons). Place the oil of rose geranium and the glycerine in the bottom and roll them round to coat the inside of the bowl. Cover with polythene film to keep in the fragrance. As they are ready, dry the rose petals to a leathery texture and add to the bowl in layers about 12 millimetres (half an inch) deep, sprinkling each layer with a teaspoon of grain alcohol. Keep the bowl in a dark, dry, airy place and cover only partially once you have started to add petals. When the potpourri is complete, toss the petals lightly with salt, cover and cure for 2 weeks, shaking gently daily. Blend remaining ingredients and toss with petals. Cover, but do not seal, and let stand 2 weeks. This recipe recommends the addition of a teaspoon of grain alcohol every time the potpourri is opened for use.

Sweet Jar, 1839

This is an old recipe adapted from *Miss Leslie's Directions for Cooking*. The salt is fine rather than coarse, and the blender and fixative is orris-root. If you cannot obtain balm of Gilead, use a musk oil sparingly. The ingredients are cured separately in 2 jars, then blended.

CROCK 1

1½ cups fresh damask roses
1½ cups petals of clove pinks
¼ cup wallflower petals
1½ cups any other fragrant
   flower
½ cup fine salt
30 g (1 oz.) orris-root sliced
   fine (about ½ cup)

CROCK 2

1 cup fresh lavender
1 cup marjoram
1 cup rosemary
1 cup thyme
1 cup balm of Gilead
1 cup lemon peel
¼ cup bay leaves
¼ cup mint leaves
1 teaspoon ground cinnamon
1 teaspoon ground clove
1 teaspoon ground nutmeg
30 g (1 oz.) orris-root sliced
   fine (about ½ cup)
½ cup fine salt

Dry the flower petals to a leathery texture. In a 3½-litre (6-pint) crock, layer the petals, covering each 12-millimetre (half-inch) layer with a little salt and sliced orris-root. Chop all the herbs finely and layer in a second crock, covering each layer with a little salt and slices of orris-root. Store both crocks, lightly covered, in a dry, airy place, and stir daily until contents are dry. Combine contents of both crocks, seal, and cure for 8 weeks. Keep potpourri sealed when not in use.

4
Dry Potpourris and the Rose Bowl

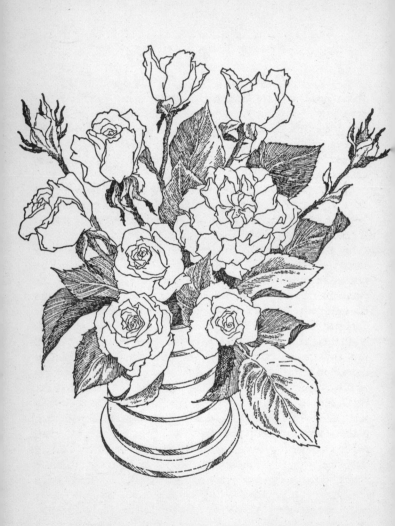

4

DRY POTPOURRIS AND
THE ROSE BOWL

ROSE petals and rosebuds are the main ingredients of a true
rose bowl, but you can capture all the flowers of summer in a
dry potpourri. Pick and dry petals as the season brings the
flowers to bloom, store them in separate containers, and when
the garden chores are over and the Christmas gift list beckons,
make them into potpourris for presents.

Pick perfect, just-opening blossoms after the dew has gone
on a dry sunny morning, but before the heat of the day has
begun to volatilize the essential oils that carry the fragrance.
Or pick them before dew falls in the early evening.

Set the petals to dry, as described in Chapter 3, but leave
them about ten days, or until they are as dry as cornflakes. You
can make up your potpourri at once, or you may store the
petals in a bone-dry container, tightly sealed and away from
the light, until the autumn when you may have more time.

Herbs can be harvested in mid-morning on a dry day. Don't
wash them as you would for cooking. Pick leaves at the branch
tips and spread them to dry, one layer deep on screens, as
described at the beginning of the last chapter for the drying
of flowers and flower petals. If you are short of time, and the
herbs are just ripe for picking – just before the buds open they
seem to have the strongest scent and flavour – pick branch tips,
gather them into small bunches, and tie them up in brown
paper bags. Hung from a clothesline in the attic, they'll dry
dust-free within two weeks. Strip the leaves gently from the
stems, store in absolutely dry containers, seal and keep away
from light until you are ready to use them.

To harvest the seeds of coriander and other herbs for potpourris, watch the seedheads closely as they begin to ripen, and

just before they are ripe, cut the whole seed stalk. Gather the stalks head down into bunches, and hang in a paper bag in a dry place. In ten days or two weeks, shake the bag and the seeds will drop to the bottom. Place the seeds in a bowl and blow gently to remove the bits of chaff mixed with them. Store them as suggested for flowers and herbs. It's a good idea to label containers of herb seeds and leaves; by the time you are ready to use them, you may not remember what is what as they all look, but don't smell, rather alike.

Because the petals and leaves for dry potpourris are completely dry before the potpourri is made – they don't 'rot' in the pot – the dry potpourri is prettier. But it is still apt to be faded in colour and look a little dusty. When mine turn out that way, I add a handful of rosebuds, dried chamomile flowers, and sometimes blue mallow petals, to improve the colour and texture of the mixture. Almost any attractive dried flower serves, so as summer waxes and wanes, pick colourful zinnias, marigolds, nasturtiums – anything the garden can spare – and dry the petals in the oven or in sand mixed half-and-half with laundry borax. Or use silica gel. Dried in these mediums they shrink, but remain whole and often retain their colour better than air-dried flowers. (I don't recommend this method for drying the bulk of the potpourri ingredients because of the space and amount of silica gel that would be required.)

Long ago in the stillrooms, flowers were dried over artificial heat for special purposes, and sometimes in sand or sugar. In *The Receipt Book of John Nott* (1723), an old recipe book by the man who was the cook to the Duke of Bolton, we were left these instructions for drying roses:

To Dry Roses

Take the Buds of Damask Roses before they are fully blown, pull the leaves and lay them on Boards, in a Room where the Heat of the Sun may not come at them; when they are pretty dry, let a large still be made warm, and lay them on the Top of it till they are crisp; but let them not lie so long as to change their Colour. Then spread them thin; and when they are thoroughly dry'd, press them down into an Earthen Pan, and keep close cover'd.

Here is Mary Doggett's recipe for drying roses.

To Dry Roses For Sweet Powder

Take your Roses after they have layen 2 or 3 days on a Table (leather dry), then put them into a dish and sett them on a chafering dish of Charcole, keeping them stirred, and as you stir them strew in some powder of orris, and when you see them pretty dry put them into a gally pot till you use them.

And here's a drying method from *The Toilet of Flora*.

To Dry Flowers

Take fine white sand, wash it repeatedly, till it contains not the least earth or salt, then dry it for use. When thoroughly dry, fill a glass or stone jar half full of Sand in which stick the Flowers in their natural situation, and afterwards cover them gently with the same, about an eighth part of an inch above the Flower.

Flora then kept the jar in the sun or in a well-warmed room until the flowers were completely dry. After removing them from their sandy bed very gently, she brushed the flowers carefully with a feather brush.

I find silica gel, which is a grainy light material sold by florists and garden-supply centres, is the fastest and best drying medium. An old dress box makes an excellent container for drying. Spread a layer of silica gel over the bottom of the box, lay the petals flat on the gel; gently sift 25 millimetres (an inch or so) of gel over them. The average dress box will take 3 to 4 layers of petals. If you are layering petals of different flowers, put the thickest on the bottom. They will take the longest to dry. Left too long in the gel, the petals become so brittle they shatter at the slightest touch, so put a set of sample petals, one of each sort, in gel in the corner of the box and check it every

two or three days to see how far along the drying process is for
each type. You can also dry whole flowers this way and glue
them onto the inside walls of plain jars intended for potpourris
– they are very pretty, although fragile.

The next two recipes appear in three variations so you can
get a feeling for how to cut ingredients when you want to
make a smaller quantity of any given recipe. An advantage in
making mini-mixtures is that you can judge how well you like
the fragrance without committing yourself to bucketsful of any
particular potpourri.

Easy Rose Potpourri

You will probably want to buy the rosebuds from the herbalist's (p. 125), rather than commit that many of your roses to
premature extinction.

3 cups dried rosebuds	½ teaspoon dried mint leaves
½ teaspoon coarse-ground cloves	½ teaspoon coarse-ground allspice
½ teaspoon coarse-ground cinnamon	1½ teaspoons ground orris-root
	3 drops oil of roses

Combine the rosebuds, spices and mint in a bowl. Mix in
the orris-root powder and the oil of roses. Seal tight, and set to
cure in a warm, dry, dark place for 6 weeks. Shake gently every
day. Transfer to small attractive containers, or to a single large
bowl with a lid. It can't be said too often that no potpourri will
retain its fragrance if it is constantly exposed to air. It must be
kept covered always, and the lid removed and the contents
stirred up just before you want to scent a room. Leave off the
lid while using the room, then re-cover the potpourri at once.

Small Rose Potpourri

The above recipe can be made up in 1- or 2-cup batches for
giving or testing. A comparison of the proportionate reduc-

tion in spices in the recipes below will help you to work out
reductions of larger recipes. Start with 2 drops of oil of roses;
add one more if you find this too faint.

2 cups dried rosebuds	½ teaspoon coarse-ground
½ teaspoon coarse-ground	allspice
cloves	½ teaspoon dried mint leaves
½ teaspoon coarse-ground	1½ teaspoons orris-root powder
cinnamon	2 or 3 drops oil of roses

Proceed as above in recipe for Easy Rose Potpourri.

Mini Rose Potpourri

1 cup dried rosebuds	¼ teaspoon coarse-ground
¼ teaspoon coarse-ground	allspice
cloves	½ teaspoon dried mint leaves
¼ teaspoon coarse-ground	¾ teaspoon orris-root powder
cinnamon	2 drops oil of roses

Proceed as in recipe for Easy Rose Potpourri. Add dried
marigold and blue mallow petals if the mixture looks unin-
teresting.

Marigold-and-Mint Potpourri

I think the purpose of the salt in a dry potpourri is more to
bulk out the contents than to improve the chemical reaction.
This mixture has a dry minty scent. Add 2 drops more of the
basil and the peppermint oils if you find the scent too faint. If
oil of basil is hard to find, increase the amount of dried basil
to 1 cupful; if oil of peppermint is unavailable, try peppermint
flavouring essence or ½ cup dry peppermint leaves.

½ cup dried thyme	½ cup dried marigold fllowers
¾ cup dried peppermint leaves	2 drops oil of peppermint
⅓ cup dried basil	2 drops oil of basil
¼ cup coarse sea salt	

Crush the herbs lightly and mix with the salt. Add the marigolds and mix in the oil of peppermint and of basil. Seal the jar, set in a dark, dry, warm place for 6 weeks, shaking once daily.

Variation on Marigold-and-Mint

A note about substitutes for oil of peppermint and oil of basil is given in the introduction to the basic recipe. The chamomile is added to vary colour and texture.

⅓ cup dried thyme	⅓ cup dried chamomile
½ cup dried peppermint leaves	½ cup dried marigold flowers
¼ cup dried basil	2 drops oil of peppermint
⅓ cup coarse sea salt	2 drops oil of basil

Proceed as for Marigold-and-Mint Potpourri.

Another Variation on Marigold-and-Mint

Like the chamomile, blue mallow flowers have been added simply to change the colour and texture of the mixture. A note about substitutes for oil of peppermint and oil of basil is given in the introduction to the basic recipe.

¼ cup dried thyme	⅓ cup dried marigold flowers
¼ cup dried peppermint leaves	2 tablespoons blue mallow
2 tablespoons of basil	flowers
¼ cup coarse salt	2 drops oil of peppermint
¼ cup dried chamomile	2 drops oil of basil

Proceed as for Marigold-and-Mint Potpourri.

Lavender Potpourri

This is a fairly traditional lavender potpourri, which would be attractive in a glass dish with a cover. The most highly scented lavender flowers are not the most deeply coloured, but if you happen to be growing some less fragrant but beautifully purple lavender in your garden, use it. This recipe relies on oil of lavender for its fragrance. You can also add dried delphinium or larkspur, or blue salvia, purple pansies or violets to give this potpourri some of the colour the fragrance leads you to expect. If you use the pale lavender buds in their natural colour, scatter a handful of red rosebuds through the mixture – the dusty tones of grey and green and the hint of pinky-red give this potpourri the charm of an old-fashioned print.

2 cups dried lavender flowers	*2 tablespoons dried sweet basil*
2 tablespoons dried lemon peel	*2 tablespoons dried rosemary*
4 tablespoons orris-root powder	*1 teaspoon gum benzoin*
4 tablespoons dried peppermint leaves	*6 drops oil of lavender*

Gently combine all ingredients except the oil. Finally add the oil, a drop at a time, tossing as you add. Seal and store in a dark, dry, warm place for 6 weeks, shaking daily.

Rose Bowl

The tonka beans, ground, have a sweetish scent like vanilla, and add a sustaining note to the fragrance of this mixture. The rose leaves bring a charming touch of faded green.

8 cups dried rose petals	*4 tablespoons coarse-ground cinnamon*
4 cups dried rose leaves	*¼ cup coarse-ground cloves*
6 cups dried lavender flowers	*4 tonka beans, ground*
⅔ cup orris-root powder	*4 drops oil of roses*
4 tablespoons coarse-ground allspice	*2 drops oil of lavender*

Gently combine all the dry ingredients. At the end, add the oils, a drop at a time, mixing as you do. Seal the jar and cure for 6 weeks in a dry, dark, warm place, shaking daily.

Potpourri from the Far East

The santal or sandalwood and patchouli leaves turn this into an Indian perfume. The patchouli leaves give a more delicate fragrance than oil of patchouli, which might be used instead. If you can't get either oakmoss or vetiver, you might like to experiment by increasing the quantity of tonka beans and adding a couple of broken cinnamon sticks; but I haven't tried it myself. This is a heavy potpourri; try a mini version before splurging.

⅓ cup orris-root powder
8 tonka beans, ground
60 g (2 oz.) ground santal or sandalwood
15 g (½ oz.) oakmoss [p. 32] or vetiver leaves
120 g (4 oz.) patchouli leaves or 10 drops patchouli oil

2 cups orange leaves or rind of ½ orange, dried, cut into tiny strips
4 cups lavender flowers
1 tablespoon ground cinnamon

Gently combine all ingredients. If you are using patchouli oil or essence in place of leaves, and find the scent too faint, add a little more, sparingly, drop by drop. Seal into a container and cure 6 weeks in a dark, dry place, shaking gently every day.

English Rose Potpourri

The gum storax called for here is available from Baldwin's (p. 125). It is difficult to work with, however, since it is very hard and has to be melted down. I suggest gum benzoin as a substitute. Alternatively, if you find oil of styrax listed, you could try that.

3 cups dried rose petals
2 cups dried lavender flowers
1 cup dried lemon verbena leaves
1 tablespoon powdered allspice

1 tablespoon coarse-ground cinnamon
1 tablespoon coarse-ground cloves
7 g (¼ oz.) gum benzoin or gum storax

Combine all dry ingredients, and add the gum storax or gum benzoin. If oil of styrax is used, add a drop at a time, mixing as you add, until the scent seems strong enough. Seal the container, and cure in a dry, dark place for 6 weeks, shaking every day.

Hungarian Potpourri

This is a variation on a popular potpourri, and very pleasant with its overtones of vetiver, an aromatic grass.

3 cups dried rosemary
1½ cups orange blossoms
1½ cups mint leaves
60 g (2 oz.) calamus [p. 66]
60 g (2 oz.) crushed vetiver
2 drops any oil of potpourri

3 cups dried yellow rose petals
Ground peel of dried lemon
1 cup dried yellow zinnia petals

Gently combine everything but the fragrant oil. Add the oil a drop at a time, mixing as you add. Seal and cure for 6 weeks in a dry, warm place, shaking the potpourri daily.

Mini Chypre Potpourri

This is adapted from a sachet recipe which is especially woodsy and nice. It's a mini recipe. Test it and triple quantities if you enjoy it. If you can't get patchouli leaves, add an extra ⅓ cup rosebuds and 3 drops oil of patchouli.

¼ cup blade mace
⅓ cup patchouli leaves
1 cup rosebuds

¾ cup shredded vetiver root
½ cup oakmoss or vanilla pods

Combine the mace, patchouli leaves, and rosebuds. Pull the vetiver and oakmoss (or vanilla pods) into small pieces and mix in. Seal and cure for 6 weeks in a dark, dry place, stirring occasionally.

Potpourri Marechale

The ambrette seeds (seeds of hibiscus) are brownish and have a musky scent. Calamus root (sweet flag), like cassia, has a cinnamon fragrance. It is available from Baldwin's but cinnamon can be used instead. If you cannot get cassia buds, try cinnamon sticks broken into small pieces or increase the coarse-ground cinnamon by 60 grammes (2 ounces).

2 cups dried chamomile flowers
120 g (4 oz.) ambrette seed
½ cup calamus or coarse-ground cinnamon
⅔ cup orris-root powder

60 g (2 oz.) cassia buds
1 cup dried orange blossoms or rose petals
½ cup ground cloves
Minced peel of 1 dried lemon rind

Combine all the ingredients, seal and cure in a dry, dark place for 6 weeks, shaking occasionally.

Potpourri with Coriander

Coriander, freshly ground, has a sweet, spicy smell, and combines with the other ingredients in this potpourri to produce a very delicate but quite exotic scent. Add more of the fragrant oils if you find the scent too delicate after curing.

6 cups dried rose petals
6 cups dried pinks or wallflowers
1½ cups orris-root powder
2 tablespoons ground cloves

1 cup ground coriander
3 drops oil of roses
30 g (1 oz.) gum benzoin or oil of styrax

Combine all ingredients but the fragrant oil. Add the oil a drop at a time, stirring as you add. Seal and cure in a dry, warm place, shaking daily, for 6 weeks.

Golden Potpourri

This golden potpourri has a lemony fragrance and is pretty in a golden bowl. Lemon balm is *Melissa officinalis*. If lemon verbena oil is not available, double the quantity of dried lemon verbena leaves and add 10 drops of lemon flavouring essence (or 10 drops of lime oil or lime fragrance).

1 cup dried lemon verbena leaves
1 cup dried lemon balm leaves
Peel of 1 dried lemon, cut into bits
1 cup dried chamomile flowers

1 cup dried forsythia flowers
1 cup dried yellow African marigold petals
⅓ cup orris-root powder
6 drops lemon verbena oil

Combine all dry ingredients, and add oil a drop at a time. Seal and cure in a dry, warm place for 6 weeks, shaking daily.

Chypre Potpourri

This is an adaptation from an early chypre sachet. Make a mini version to see if you like it. The fragrance is definitely exotic.

120 g (4 oz.) oakmoss [p. 32] or vetiver
2 cups rose petals
30 g (1 oz.) rosebuds
250 g (8 oz.) orange blossoms
⅔ cup coarse-ground cardamom seeds

60 g (2 oz.) sandalwood
¼ cup coarse-ground cloves
45 g (1½ oz.) gum benzoin
4 drops bitter almond oil or 4 drops almond food flavouring

Pull the oakmoss or vetiver to bits; mix in all dried ingredients well. Add oil, a drop at a time, stirring as you add. Seal and cure for 6 weeks, in a dry, dark place, shaking daily.

Old English Rose Bowl

This is one of the nicest potpourris, but quite expensive. Try a mini version to see if it suits your taste.

7 cups dried rose petals
1 cup dried rosebuds
2 cups orris-root powder
30 g (1 oz.) sandalwood
  raspings
3.5 ml (⅛ fl. oz.) oil of roses
7 ml (¼ fl. oz.) oil of
  rose geranium or ½ cup
  dried rose geranium leaves

3.5 ml (⅛ fl. oz.) oil of
  sandalwood
14 ml (½ fl. oz.) oil of bergamot
14 ml (½ fl. oz.) oil of musk

Mix roses, orris-root powder and sandalwood raspings and add oils a little at a time, stirring as you add. Mix the whole well, then seal and cure in a dry, dark, warm room for 6 weeks, stirring or shaking the container daily so the oils blend well.

American Potpourri

Use any dried garden flowers the season yields. The hydrangea and Queen Anne's lace should be broken into florets; do not use whole heads.

1 cup dried blue salvia
1 cup dried red salvia
1 cup dried blue hydrangea
  blossoms
1 cup dried rose petals
1 cup dried pinks
1 cup dried Queen Anne's
  lace
10 drops oil of bergamot or
  120 g (4 oz.) orange
  peel, dried and pounded
  to a powder

20 drops eucalyptus oil
4 drops oil of roses
½ teaspoon coarse-ground
  cloves
⅓ cup orris-root powder
¼ teaspoon cinnamon
⅓ teaspoon coarse-ground
  mace

Gently combine all the dried flowers, then turn into a very large bowl and mix in the spices and fragrant oils, a drop at a time. Stir as you add. Seal and cure for 6 weeks in a warm, dry, dark place.

Peacock Potpourri

If you haven't all the flowers mentioned, substitute others whose colours are similar; each has been selected primarily for colour. The fragrance comes from the oils added at the end, and also from the spices and orris powder. All the petals must be completely dry.

1 cup pink rose petals
2 cups red rose petals
1 cup yellow rose petals
2 cups lavender blossoms
1 cup rose delphinium petals
1 cup blue delphinium petals
1 cup blue larkspur
1 cup blue cornflowers
1 cup yellow calendula
1 cup orange calendula
1 cup purple violets

1 cup yellow pansies
1 cup scented geranium leaves
1 cup lemon verbena leaves
1 rounded tablespoon orris-root powder
1 teaspoon ground cloves
1 teaspoon ground nutmeg
1 teaspoon ground cinnamon
8 drops any potpourri essence or essence of rose, or essence of gardenia

Gently combine flowers. Mix orris powder and spices and toss with flowers. Add the fragrant oil, a drop at a time, mixing well. Seal and cure 6 weeks. Transfer to decorative little containers of clear glass, or display in a very large punch-bowl that has a cover.

5
Sharp Fragrances: The Stillroom Way to Good Health

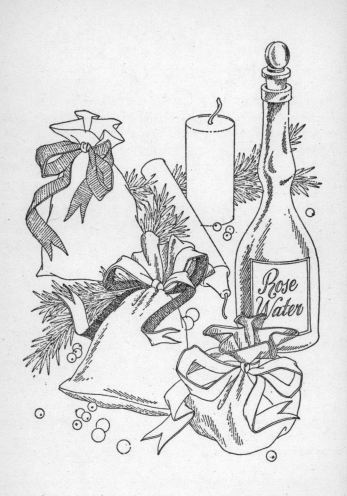

SHARP FRAGRANCES:
THE STILLROOM WAY
TO GOOD HEALTH

HERBAL fragrances are dry and sharp, but sweet, like the scent of the plants in hot sunshine. The stillroom ladies, and the Romans and Greeks before them, associated sharp fragrances with good health. And may not have been so far off. Experiments at the Pasteur Institute in Paris in the last century seem to prove that the bacilli of certain diseases prevalent in the Middle Ages – tuberculosis and various fevers – are destroyed by the essential oils in plants with sharp fragrances, such as rosemary and cloves.

Some of the stillroom ways with disinfectants and health preservatives are lovely, but not all are practical for the modern homemaker. The strewing herbs intrigue me most. I am fascinated by the idea of strewing fragrant meadowsweet and flowers all over the kitchen tiles, but appalled at the mess they would make of the rest of the house. However, tussie-mussies and wash balls and scented vinegars and perfumes to burn are easy to make and charming gifts for friends who love flowers and herbs and the romance of old-fashioned things.

The essential elements in the disinfectants made by the stillroom ladies were the herbs. Before Marco Polo and other travelling salesmen of the period reintroduced the spices and aromatics of the Far East to the West, herbs were almost all that was left to us of the fragrant ways of Egypt and Rome and Greece.

The way men and women lived in the thirteenth century as Europe moved towards the Renaissance was very different from the life-style current when Rome and Greece flourished.

In the dark years of the Middle Ages, a remnant of culture

survived in the courts of Europe and in the monasteries, but only the bare essentials for life existed in the homes of the people. Where the open atrium of Rome faced onto a court-yard heady with the scent of herbs, the cottages and castles of the colder lands had few windows or doors, the floors were beaten earth or stone, and air circulation was designed to keep fresh air out because there was no central heating. Cleaning establishments did not exist; clothes and the heavy handwoven linens were washed rarely. The kings bathed not too often, and the people less. City streets were narrow and were used as open sewers. A morning chore was to throw the night slops from the upstairs window. The stench was frightful, and as the cities became more populated, plagues haunted them and the adjacent countryside.

Beset on one hand by plagues, and on the other by the threat of 'worms in the belly and ears', by scabies, by 'dirty, filfy beasts in the clothes' and lice on the head, and by the simple discomfort of unpleasant smells on all sides, the mistress of the medieval household struggled with the help of the ancient herbals towards cleanliness and better sanitation, towards good smells that 'do make the heart merrie'.

In medieval monasteries, monks planted sweet-smelling herbs for the benefit of their patients, and cottage gardens followed suit. The stillroom ladies grew rue and rosemary against plagues, myrtle against 'joints that are loosened and fractures that are hard to grow together', chamomile to 'break the stone' and take away 'the aching of a man's head and for the megrim [migraine]'.

STREWING HERBS

Of the many uses to which herbs were put then, the strewing herb is one that has no exact modern counterpart, unless it is an aerosol spray combined with a good scrubbing with lye.

Strewing herbs date from antiquity and go through the history of England and colonial America. In antiquity, flowers and herbs were strewn primarily for the pleasure of the guests. Romans imported roses from Egypt and strewed petals on banquet floors. During the late years of the Empire, the images of Cupid, Venus and Bacchus were covered with petals; petals and herbs were scattered in processions to Flora and Hymen, victors and chariots were showered with them, and petals adorned the prows of war vessels. The strewing of palms before Jesus as he advanced into Jerusalem on Palm Sunday is a biblical reference to the practice. In English history the emphasis is on strewing herbs for sanitary reasons. In his book *500 Points of Good Husbandry*, written in 1573, Thomas Tusser, later a member of the court of James I, listed twenty-one herbs to grow for strewing, and long before the records of the Crusades the custom existed of covering floors with sweet rushes and dry flowers.

Hyssop was one of Tusser's favourite strewing herbs, and woodruff with its scent of new-mown hay was a favourite in both England and America, though the colonials were partial to rosemary and thyme as well. Elizabeth I preferred meadow-sweet, and according to Parkinson, an important herbalist of the time, all her floors were strewn with it.

Bay leaves, which had crowned Roman victors, were used by the English housewife for strewing, and the rush of the sweet flag was a favourite, particularly of Cardinal Wolsey, young Henry VIII's friend. One of the accusations against the Cardinal was an extravagant use of sweet flag, which grows in England only in certain fenlands and was costly and hard to get.

In the sixteenth century, sweet rushes were used not only on floors but also under church pews, and sometimes flowers were strewn through the pews when church services were over. Strewing was a fixed part of the cost of the crowning of kings and queens until Edward VII discontinued the practice. But throughout the nineteenth century at English coronations one lady-in-waiting was in charge of strewing herbs and with securing as many helpers as needed. For George IV there were twelve baskets, each containing two bushels of herbs and flowers, the helpers holding them high above their heads. The strewers were dressed in white muslin with flowered ornaments, and three large baskets of flowers were brought into the cathedral and placed near the ladies. At the coronation of James II, his progress along 1,220 yards of blue broadcloth was strewed with six bushels by 'The Strewer of Herbs in Ordinary to His Majesty, assisted by Six Women'.

Bunches of fragrant herbs were hung in homes and churches as decoration and to make the air sweet. Sweet woodruff was often tied with lavender and used to decorate churches, a practice that existed in colonial America as well as in sixteenth-century England. In his *Herball* (1597) Gerard wrote of woodruff '. . . being made into garlands or bundles and hanged up in the house in the heat of the day, both very well attemper the aire, coole and make fresh the place, to the delight and comfort of such that are therein.' Yarrow was used in colonial America for the same purpose.

The only modern equivalent would be the use of scented oils for floors and furniture, a custom that is recorded in the early seventeenth century. When James I visited the Bodleian Library at Oxford in the early seventeenth century, the floors had been rubbed with fresh rosemary, and oil of lavender was used on the furniture.

Some of the Elizabethans' love for garlands of flowers and herbs for strewing is recorded in the 'Wedding Song' in Edmund Spenser's *Epithalamion* (1595).

> And let them also with them bring in hand,
> Another gay girland
> For my fayre love of lillyes and of roses,
> Bound truelove wize with a blew silk riband.
> And let them make great store of bridal poses,
> And let them eeke bring store of other flowers
> To deck the bridale bowers.
> And let the ground whereas her foot shall tread,
> For feare the stones her tender foot should wrong
> Be strewed with fragrant flowers all along,
> And diapered lyke the discoloured mead.

The Elizabethans' infinite faith in the magic of flowers and herbs is clear in this recipe, dated 1600 and now in the Ashmolean Museum in Oxford.

To Enable One to See Fairies

A pint of sallet oyle and put it into a vial glasse; and first wash it with rose-water and marygold water; the flowers to be gathered towards the east. Wash it till the oyle becomes white, then put into the glasse, and then put thereto the budds of holly-hocke, the flowers of marygolde, the flowers or toppes of wild thyme, the budds of young hazle, and the thyme must be gathered near the side of a hill where fairies used to be; and take the grasse of a fairy throne; then all these put into the oyle in the glasse and sette it to dissolve 3 dayes in the sunne and keep it for thy use.

It is still pleasant on a hot summer day to pick a bunch of any of these herbs. Hung in a corner of the dining room, they bring a faint fragrance to the evening air. I've tried scrubbing floors with bunches of fresh lavender – too extravagant a gesture for my small supply of this precious fragrance – and with rosemary, and the spicy scent lasts well. Most rewarding because they last longer are some of the many other stillroom products made with fragrant herbs.

Gather the herbs before the dew dries on a dry day; pick the leafy tips, and if possible plan to harvest just before the flower buds bloom.

TUSSIE-MUSSIES

An interesting historical use of herbs was the tussie-mussie, a nosegay of selected herbs sometimes interspersed with flowers. John Parkinson names these little bouquets in his *Paradisus*, written in 1629. Each flower and herb used had a specific meaning that most medieval and Elizabethan men and women knew well. (See Chapter 7, Table F, for a list of a few of the best-known ones.) The tussie-mussie itself conveyed a special meaning, usually romantic, although its origin must have been medicinal. The first tussie-mussies were probably little bunches of rue and other herbs carried to combat the unpleasant odours of bad sanitation and to fight off plague germs.

The Colonials favoured rosemary in their herb bouquets, and sprigs of it were often tied to wedding bouquets as a symbol of remembrance. When valentines came into fashion, a sprig of rosemary was often painted on a heart and sent to the object of one's affections. This kind of remembrance was extended to sadder occasions: at funerals each mourner left a sprig on the coffin. In England, gilded branches or rosemary tied with ribbons were given to wedding guests and brides-maids wore sprigs of it on the left arm to symbolize faithful-ness. Elizabeth II was handed a tussie-mussie as she entered Westminster Abbey on the day of her coronation.

The colonists were fond of forget-me-nots, also a symbol of faithfulness and remembrance, and forget-me-nots were often given to people starting on a journey on 29 February. Later on the forget-me-nots were mixed with various herbs that had special meanings, and these little tussie-mussies were given to friends on 29 February. The whole concept of a bouquet that makes a sentimental statement appealed to the romantic imagination of the eighteenth century and there are many references to the custom in literature.

Shakespeare had a complete fragrant garden and put a lot of herbal lore into his plays. In *Hamlet*, Act IV, scene v, after the killing of Ophelia's father, the daughter puts together a tussie-mussie that carries a tragic, bitter little message:

> There's rosemary, that's for remembrance;
> pray you, love, remember; and there is
> pansies, that's for thoughts.
> There's fennel for you, and columbines;
> there's rue for you; and here's some for
> me; we may call it herb of grace o'
> Sundays; O, you must wear your rue with a
> difference. There's a daisy; I would
> give you some violets but they withered all
> when my father died.

(Fennel stood for flattery, dissembling; columbines for unchastity; rue for repentance, contrition and grief; when mixed with holy water it was known as 'herb of grace'. Daisies stood for wantonness, faithlessness; and violets, when blue, were for loyalty, when white, for innocence.)

More cheerful combinations for tussie-mussies of the past were marigolds and heartsease, coupled to mean happiness and remembrance; sage and chamomile, to wish a friend longevity, sagacity, and patience. Marjoram and lily-of-the-valley in a tussie-mussie were symbols of purity, happiness, and humility.

Tussie-mussies from your garden make charming gifts. They will last for years if the herbs and flowers are dried in silica gel. The scent of a dried tussie-mussie is faint – stronger if the day is humid or particularly warm – but you can bring it up a little by tying the bouquet with a ribbon that has been steeped in cologne and then dried. Use grosgrain, which stands soaking best. Or after the nosegay is made up, but at least two weeks before it is to be given, use an eyedropper to deposit one or two drops of a suitable floral essence onto stems in the interior of the bouquet, and 'cure' the tussie-mussie in a sealed brown paper bag away from the light.

Use the Language of the Plants (Table F, Chapter 7) to make sure your tussie-mussie says what you want it to say. When I make one as a gift, I include a note explaining the meaning of the flowers and herbs in the bouquet.

BURNING PERFUMES

The use of burning perfumes, incense, to disinfect and make fragrant rooms and people is as old as the Bible and is still practised among nomadic tribes of the Near East. The Macedonian who created the Greek empire of classical times, Alexander the Great, picked up the habit during his eastern campaigns, and the Roman housewife used censers to fumigate her apartments, too. The English borrowed the practice, which was common until after the reign of Henry VIII's only son, Edward VI (1547–53). It is tempting to guess that the use of incense declined because it was associated with the Roman church which Edward repudiated.

Several recipes for burning perfumes have been left to us. One favoured by Edward VI was a boiling perfume. Here is a later recipe:

Boiling Perfume

12 spoonfuls of bright red rose-water, the weight of 6 pence in fine powder sugar, and boil it on hot embers and coals softly, and the room will smell as though it were full of roses; but you must burn sweet cyprus wood before, to take away the gross air.

The Queen's Closet, 1662

Here are others to try; they have come to us from the sixteenth, seventeenth, and eighteenth centuries.

A Perfume for the Chamber

Take of Storax [double the benzoin as a substitute], Calamint [related to savory; try mint or savory or basil leaves as a substitute], Benzoin, Aloes Wood, of each 1 oz. [30 grammes], Coales [ashes] of Willow, well beaten in to powder, 5 oz. [150 grammes]. These things mixed with Aqua Vitae, as much as will make a paste. Make thereof little cakes, or other forms if you will, and so keep them. And when you will use or occupy it, put it into a fire, for in consuming little by little, it will make a singular good odour in the place where you burn it.

The Secrets of Alexis, 1555

Perfumed Incense to Burn

Take 2 oz. [60 grammes] of the Powder of Juniper Wood, 1 oz. [30 grammes] of Benjamin, 1 oz. Storax [double the benzoin as a substitute], 6 drops of oil of Lemons, as much oil of Cloves, 10 grains of Musk [try 5 drops essence of musk, adding more if you wish], 6 of them in little Cakes and dry them between Rose leaves, your juniper wood must be well dried, beaten and searced [sieved].

The Queen's Closet, 1662

To Perfume a House, and Purify the Air

Take a root of Angelica, dry it in an oven, or before the fire, then bruise it well and infuse it 4 or 5 days in White Wine Vinegar. When you use it, lay it upon a brick made red hot, and repeat the operation several times.

The Toilet of Flora, 1775

Nineteenth-century instructions for a burning perfume begin with a quarter of a pound [120 grammes] of damask roses, beaten to a mash, and mixed with a third of a cup of orris-root powder soaked in a quarter of a cup of rose water. The whole is combined, 5 grains of musk and 2 ounces [60 grammes] of powdered gum benzoin are added, then some sugar to absorb any remaining moisture. If the mixture is too dry to absorb any sugar, add a few drops or rose water. The perfume is then formed into small cakes which are set on paper in the direct sun to dry for a few days. Burn the cakes on lighted charcoal – ideally the perfumers' charcoal that is used for the burning of incense – or else on glowing but flameless coals from the fireplace.

A burning perfume popular in the Middle Ages is based on the old biblical use, blending one part myrrh to 5 parts frankincense, to 2½ parts benzoin. The whole is mixed and burned on charcoal.

Any of the fixatives for potpourris make nice burning perfumes. My favourites are musk crystals, myrrh, sandalwood, vetiver. An attractive mixture is cassia bark, myrrh, musk, sandalwood powder, and benzoin, about equal parts blended, and burned on charcoal.

Sir Hugh Platt, in his *Delights for Ladies* (1594) suggests two or three drops of ambergris, aloes, *Lignum rhodium* (rose wood), or storax, blended and burned on charcoal.

HERBAL VINEGARS

The most popular disinfectants both in England and in colonial America were herbal vinegars. Made of many different garden herbs, they were used to ward off plague germs, to perfume sickrooms, and to improve poor ventilation. During plague epidemics, rosemary was especially in demand, and the price would skyrocket from an armful for a shilling to eightpence for a tiny bundle. Rue was believed efficacious, and rue and pitch were both burned in the streets.

In the seventeenth century, vinegars were used to soak sponges, which could be sniffed if you felt ill, and to bathe an aching brow and refresh feverish hands. The heads of walking canes were equipped with compartments holding vinegar-soaked sponges. These kept foul odours at bay as gentlemen walked in the streets and were used by doctors making their rounds of sick patients. During epidemics, men and women washed their hands and faces in the vinegars and sprinkled them over linens and bedclothes.

In time the aromatic vinegars went into vinaigrettes, which Victorian ladies wore on chains around their necks. That was the time when a lady, laced to her chin, fainted readily, and the vinaigrette's sharp scent revived her.

These herbal vinegars were not on the whole intended to be taken internally, though today vinegars are used for making salads and the method of making them is much the same.

An intriguing disinfectant is the Vinegar of the Four Thieves, which was used in England and in colonial America as well. Tradition has it that thieves intent on robbing plague victims protected themselves by sprinkling their prey and his belongings with the lotion.

Here's a Virginia housewife's 1856 version of this.

Vinegar of the Four Thieves

Take lavender, rosemary, sage, wormword, rue, and mint, of each a large handful, put them in a pot of earthenware, pour on them 4 qts [4½ litres] strong vinegar, cover the pot closely, and put a board on top; keep it in the hottest sun 2 weeks, then strain and bottle it, putting in each bottle a clove of garlic; when it has settled and become clear, pour it off gently; do this until you get it all free from sediment. The proper time to make it is when the herbs are in full vigour, in June. The vinegar is very refreshing in crowded places, in the apartments of the sick and is peculiarly grateful when sprinkled about the house in damp weather.

Alice Cooke Brown,
Early American Herb Recipes, 1966

This next vinegar, from *The Good Housewife's Jewel* (1585), was intended for internal use.

A Preventive Against Plague

A handful each of rue, sage, sweet-brier, and elder. Bruise and strain with a quart [generous 1 litre] of white wine, and put thereto a little ginger and a spoonful of the best treacle, and drink thereof morning and evening.

Another recipe for a disinfectant vinegar comes to us from *The Toilet of Flora* in the eighteenth century.

Vinegar

Handful of rosemary, wormwood, lavender, and mint to be put into a jar with a gallon [4½ litres] of strong vinegar, keep near a fire for 4 days, strain, an oz. [30 grammes] of powder camphor added and then bottled for pleasure.

You can give any vinegar the taste and fragrance of a herb; and though this book deals primarily with herbs for scent, I can't skip by herb vinegars without explaining how those we use today for flavouring salads are made. It's so easy! Just buy good white vinegar or cider vinegar, in a medium-sized bottle – about 13 fluid ounces, or 37 centilitres in metric terms – empty out about a quarter of the contents, and add four full-leafed sprigs from the tip of a herb plant. Tarragon vinegar is delicious in salads. Thyme is nice in dressings for fish salads. Dill is excellent with cold pork and in potato salad.

Mint vinegars were enormously popular in colonial America. They were used for iced tea, in fruit punches, and to make mint sauce. Here's a mint vinegar recipe that shows another method for making herb vinegars. This method calls for boiling, and I find the result has a sharper flavour. The method can be used for making any type of culinary herb vinegar, but omit the sugar and substitute one cup of bruised herb leaves.

Colonial Mint Vinegar

2 cups, packed, spearmint
1 cup granulated sugar

Generous 1 litre (1 qt)
cider vinegar

Pick tips of spearmint, wash lightly, dry without bruising. Combine with the sugar. Bring the vinegar to the boiling point; remove from the heat; pour over the sugar and the mint. With a wooden spoon, stir and press the herb leaves. Marinate in a warm room 10 days, shaking daily. Strain and bottle with a fresh mint leaf inside each bottle.

HERBS FOR THE BATH

Herb vinegars were also used to scent baths – and make them antiseptic. All sorts of other delightful herbal concoctions were made for bath water.

Attractively packaged herbal bath colognes, perfumes and vinegars are charming and inexpensive mementoes to give and are pretty to place in guest bathrooms.

Here are some recipes.

Herb Bath Bags

2 tablespoons medium-ground oatmeal

1 tablespoon dry mixed herbs (rosemary, chamomile, crumbled bay leaf, thyme, basil, combined according to personal tastes)

Put ingredients in muslin or doubled cheesecloth bag. Swish bag in hot water before bathing. Can be used twice.

Bath Vinegar

1 cup cider vinegar
1 cup water

1 tablespoon dried basil
2 tablespoons dried peppermint

Combine vinegar and water; heat until nearly boiling. Remove heat and add herbs. (You can experiment with your own combinations.) Let steep overnight. Strain liquid off carefully into a jar. Allow 1 cup for the bath.

Bath Cologne

½ cup fresh fragrant rose petals
½ cup 70-proof alcohol
2 tablespoons lemon peel
1 tablespoon orange peel

1 tablespoon dried basil
1 tablespoon dried peppermint
1 cup boiling water

Soak rose petals in alcohol for 6 days in a tightly closed jar. On the fifth day steep lemon peel, orange peel, basil and peppermint in 1 cup of boiling water; cover and let stand overnight. The next day strain the liquid through cheesecloth or a nylon stocking until clear. Drain alcohol from rose petals. Combine the 2 liquids in a jar and cover tightly. Shake well. Use as after-bath cologne.

Ben Jonson thought well of bath herbs, and offers this far-fetched recipe in *Volpone, or The Fox*, Act III, scene ii:

> If thou hast wisdom, hear me, Celia.
> Thy baths shall be the juice of July-flowers,
> Spirit of Roses, and of violets,
> The milk of unicorns, and panthers' breath
> Gathered in bags and mixed with Cretan wines.

Easier to come by are the ingredients in the early recipes given below. These were meant to soothe edgy nerves and relax strained heads and sore feet.

Perfumed Bath

Take of Roses, Citron flowers, Orange flowers, Jasmine, Bay, Rosemary, Lavender, Mint, Pennyroyal and Citron peel, each of sufficient quantity, boyl them together gently, and make a bath, to which add Oyl of Spike 6 drops, Musk 5 grains, Ambergrease 3 grains, Sweet Asa 1 oz. [30 grammes]. Let her go into the Bath before meat.

C. J. S. Thompson,
The Mystery and Lure of Perfume, 1927

Colonial Bath Mix

Flowers of chamomile, leaves of peppermint, sage, rosemary, and thyme all dried first and then sewed up in a cheesecloth bag to be dropped into the bath.

C. J. S. Thompson,
The Mystery and Lure of Perfume, 1927

Here is Flora's recipe for sore feet.

Aromatic Foot Bath

Take 4 handfuls of pennyroyal, sage, rosemary, 3 handfuls of angelica and 4 ounces [120 grammes] juniper berries; boil these ingredients in a sufficient quantity of water and strain off the liquid for use.

The Toilet of Flora, 1775

HERB TEAS

Herb teas were the panacea for many ills from the Middle Ages on, and they are still favoured in Europe today. I can recall with pleasure the mint teas my mother administered for stomach aches, and I give them to my own children (and to anyone else who will submit) for an upset stomach. Many modern herb teas are held in high repute. The first recipe on the facing page is fairly standard, the other two are recipes from Linda Huntington, a herb enthusiast.

Linda believes firmly – and she is an energetic person – that herb teas aid digestion, provide a tonic effect, and soothe cold-sufferers. She sweetens her teas with honey, often adding a little lemon or orange peel or a bit of crushed cinnamon, clove, or nutmeg. She never uses milk with herb tea. Her basic method for making teas of caraway, dill, fennel, anise, thyme, or what you will, is to add one teaspoon of the herb, slightly bruised, per cup of boiling water, and she always brews in earthenware or glass pots. Water just comes to the boil; and tea steeps at least ten minutes.

Rosehip–Hibiscus Tea

Rosehip tea is reputed to be the most beneficial of herb teas and it can be drunk several times a day. Most people have to get used to the rather sharp flavour of this tea, even after sweetening with honey.

¼ cup seeded rosehips   ¼ cup dried hibiscus flowers

Clean any debris from the hibiscus flowers and combine with the rosehips. Allow 1 teaspoon of tea to 1 cup of water and brew about 20 minutes.

Rosehips are a rich source of vitamin C and are supposed to help the gall bladder and kidneys to function properly. The hibiscus flowers give a rich burgundy colour to the tea and a slightly tart lemon taste. Use honey to sweeten to taste.

Linda's Lemon Balm Tea

This tea has a mild sedative effect. It can be drunk at night to ease and soothe nerves. Serve with a little honey. This is a good tea for your first try – the herb taste is slight. A good pick-me-up in the morning too. Use 1 teaspoon per cup and let steep at least 10 minutes. Lemon balm tea is supposed to prolong life by alleviating tension and sharpening mental faculties!

2 cups dried lemon balm	*1 cup orange blossoms*
1 cup rosebuds	

Lemon balm is a twiggy herb and must be cleaned carefully. Strip leaves from all twigs. Crush the leaves slightly; add rosebuds and orange flowers, and mix well.

Chamomile Mint Tea

Peppermint is more pungent than other members of the mint family. It is a good pick-me-up for fatigue, aids digestion, and is a substitute for coffee for those with gall-bladder trouble. Chamomile flowers also aid digestion, making this a good after-dinner tea.

1 cup dry peppermint leaves	*½ cup chamomile flowers*

Blend ingredients, mixing well. Use one teaspoon of the herb mixture per cup and steep at least 10 minutes.

Mother's Mint Tea

Mint tea mixed with regular tea, half-and-half, and iced, is a refreshing drink for a hot day. Add a bit of lemon.

5 tablespoons dried peppermint leaves	*5 cups boiling water*
	2 teaspoons granulated sugar

Scald the teapot and put in the mint leaves. Bring 5 cups of fresh water to a rapid boil, and pour over the mint. Add the sugar. Steep 10 minutes. Stir up the leaves and the sugar, then pour through a strainer into serving cups. Add a bit more sugar for guests with a sweet tooth.

HERB PILLOWS

Herb pillows are small fragrant accessories, especially lovely in needlepoint or crewel-work pillow slips or covers. In time the fragrance fades, so leave one corner of your pillow loosely stitched. Then you can revive the fragrance by adding a few drops of essential oil to the mixture inside.

Herb pillows, historically, are an extension of the custom of stuffing mattresses with fragrant grasses – a common practice before the days of goosedown, horsehair, and foam rubber. The Romans filled mattresses with fragrant grasses mixed with rose petals. Lady's bedstraw, *Galium verum*, preferred in Elizabethan times, was loved for its fresh, grassy scents. Sometimes it was mixed with lavender. Charles VI of France, in the fourteenth century, sat on lavender-stuffed pillows so as to be surrounded by his favourite scent. And we catch a glimpse of Shakespeare's view of what made for sound sleep in Oberon's speech from *A Midsummer Night's Dream*, Act II, scene i:

> I know a bank where the wild thyme blows,
> Where oxlips and the nodding violet grows,
> Quite overcanopied with lush woodbine,
> With sweet musk-roses and with eglantine.
> There sleeps Titania sometime of the night,
> Lulled in these flowers with dances and delight ...

Here are Linda Huntington's three favourite herb pillow mixtures. They are meant to make small, fragrant pillows to slip under your sleeping pillow at night. If you wrap the scent pillow in your nightclothes in the morning and tuck the nightclothes under the bed pillow, you'll have fragrant nightclothes, as well as fragrant air, to sleep with.

Herb Pillows

1 tablespoon crushed whole cloves	*½ cup dried rosemary*
	1 cup dried marjoram
1 crushed cinnamon stick	*¼ cup dried spearmint*

1 *teaspoon ground allspice*
1 *teaspoon cardamom seed*
¼ *dry rind of medium-sized lemon*
1 *cup dried lavender*
½ *cup dried lemon thyme*

1 *tablespoon crushed orris-root*
1 *tablespoon gum benzoin*
5 *drops essence of bergamot or 60 g (2 oz.) orange peel dried and pounded to powder*

Alternate layers of spices and herbs and sprinkle each with a little orris, gum benzoin, and bergamot. Repeat this procedure until all ingredients are used. Store in a tightly covered box for 6 to 8 weeks. Fill cotton or silk bags to put under sleeping pillows.

Rosemary Herb Pillows

1 *cup dried rosemary leaves*
1 *cup dried lemon verbena leaves*

2 *cups dried pine needles*

Slightly crush and blend ingredients. Fill small bags to put under sleeping pillows.

Floral Herb Pillows

1 *cup dried fragrant roses*
1 *cup other dried fragrant flowers*
1 *cup dried lavender*
1 *cup dried lemon verbena*

1 *cup dried rosemary*
6 *drops essence of bergamot or 70 g (2½ oz.) orange peel dried and pounded to powder*

Combine dried flowers and herbs, and mix in the bergamot essence. Fill little silk bags to put under bed pillow.

6
Sweet Bags and
Pomanders

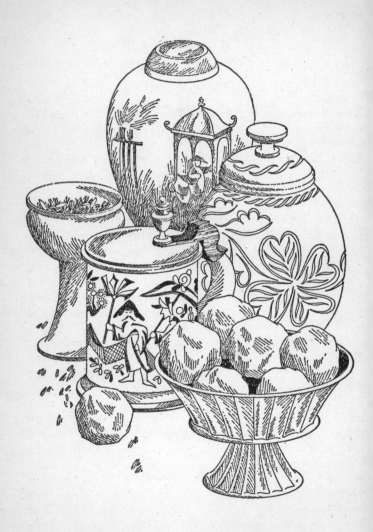

6

SWEET BAGS AND
POMANDERS

By the 1200s, the warlike life-style of the Middle Ages had mellowed and in castle and cottage garden alike there grew plants for pleasure as well as those meant to battle illness. Raised flower borders appeared and there were topiaries and fountains. Chamomile grew along the pathways and released its spicy scent when trodden on. Fragrant little clipped hedges of lavender, sage, rosemary and southernwood became popular. During the Elizabethan age, mazes were developed, and labyrinths, parterres and knot gardens with ribbon outlines of herbs. There were statues and vases and sundials, and finally – a gift of the adventurous sea captains – daffodils, fritillarias, hyacinths, crocuses, lilies, tulips, anemones, cowslips, and snapdragons, the purely ornamental flowers, found their way from far corners to European gardens. In the stillrooms, spices and exotic fixatives multiplied.

But even during the years when the Elizabethan housewife struggled with herbs and salves in her stillroom, and the colonial American grew her medicines in the backyard, the courts and courtiers of Europe, with better access to valuable ingredients, carried on the fragrant traditions of Rome and Greece and Egypt. In the eighth century, Charlemagne, trying to recreate the great days of Rome in a still-primitive Europe, used rose water lavishly, and there were professional perfumers in Paris as early as 1190.

During the Crusades, through contact with the pleasure-loving courts of the East, an interest in fragrance for its own sake was re-awakened in Europe. By the time Philip II of France came to power late in the twelfth century, perfumers were being granted charters, and when Charles the Wise took over, acres of flowers were grown to produce fragrant materials.

Perfumes distilled from alcohol – colognes – appeared in the 1300s, but dry fragrances made from the materials we use today in potpourris were more common, and they were used for various purposes. With the increase in culture in Europe in the thirteenth and fourteenth centuries, the uses of perfume multiplied, and by the seventeenth century almost everything was scented, from gloves to ink.

The first alcoholic perfume recorded was in 1370. This was a recipe given to Queen Elizabeth of Hungary; its purpose was to keep her beautiful, and it must have worked because she landed the King of Poland when she was in her seventies. The perfume, called Hungary Water, was made by distilling 1 gallon of grain alcohol with 2 ounces of otto (attar, the purest, strongest form) of rosemary, 1 ounce of otto of lemon-scented balm (*Melissa officinalis*), another of lemon peel, ½ drachma of otto of mint, and 1 pint each of extract of roses and orange blossoms.

Carmelite water was the next alcoholic distillation to attract attention. The concoction called for ½ gallon of orange-blossom water, 1 gallon of alcohol, 2 pounds of fresh balm leaves, ¼ pound of lemon peel, 2 ounces of nutmeg, 2 ounces of cloves, 2 ounces of coriander seeds, 1 ounce of cinnamon, and 1 ounce of angelica root, all of this distilled.

Preferences for fragrance of one kind or another were associated with certain personages, and through the records of the courts we catch a glimpse of the scents that were developed for them. Diane de Poitiers, who was mistress to Francis I in the 1500s and later to Henry II, was a patroness of perfume; Henry III had his linens scented with sachets of violet-scented orris-root powder, dried leaves of fragrant red roses, sandalwood, benjamin, storax, calamus root, cloves, ambergris, coriander, and lavender. Cardinal Richelieu perfumed his rooms by blowing with a bellows a scented powder of roses, cypress root, marjoram, cloves, benjamin, storax. Louis XIV loved sheets made fragrant with aloes, nutmeg, cloves, storax benzoin boiled in rose water and combined with orange flowers, jasmine, and a little musk. Marie Antoinette, the extravagant wife of Louis XVI, preferred the natural fragrances of roses and violets.

Napoleon and Josephine used scents lavishly. Josephine's room was heady with musk – which Napoleon disliked. Napoleon's preference was for sharp scents from herbs native to southern France and to his home in Corsica. He used soap scented with rosemary, otto of caraway, thyme, and clove. During his Egyptian campaign he discovered the violet-scented mignonette and sent plants back to Josephine, who adored violets. His delight in cologne has been called 'almost suspect', because the records show that he used as many as sixty bottles a month of eau de cologne.

There's a sad little flower story related to these two ill-fated lovers. Napoleon had his marriage to the lovely Creole annulled and she retired to Malmaison and died there four years later. Napoleon covered her grave with violets, and shortly before his final exile he picked violets from the grave and put them into a locket. He wore this on a chain around his neck until his death.

Pomanders and scented candles, fragrant inks and wash balls, perfumed beads and perfumed books are a few of the sweet-smelling things left to us from these centuries. Some are fun to experiment with and others make life more gracious. The sachet, or sweet bag, is perhaps the most useful of all.

SACHETS AND SWEET BAGS

From the days of Elizabeth I, rich and poor alike made sweet bags with which to scent the everyday things of life; they were placed in drawers, among linens, in the bookshelves in the library, carried in clothes, tied to chair-backs.

The most common herbs for sweet bags and pads were – along with rose petals, rosemary and marjoram – basil, thyme, coriander, anise, and caraway, and, of course, lavender flowers. The spices and fixatives were those for potpourris – cinnamon, clove, nutmeg, orris-root powder, benjamin – but the composition was different and the scent headier, since the mixtures were enclosed in fabric. Here is a recipe from our stillroom lady of the seventeenth century, Mary Doggett, along with some recipes from other centuries. Where no instructions are given, ingredients are simply to be dried, combined and poured into small muslin or silk bags. In early recipes, rose 'leaves' usually means rose petals.

Sweet Bag

A bag to smell unto for Melancholy or to cause one to sleep. Take drie Rose leaves, keep them close in a glasse which will keep them sweet, then take powder of Mints, powder of Cloves in grosse powder, and put the same to the Rose leaves, then put all these together in a bag, and take that to bed with you, and it will cause you to sleep, and it is good to smell unto at other times.

Mary Doggett,
Her Book of Recipes, 1682

Sweetbag

Take of Orris 6 oz., of Damask Rose-leaves as much, of Marjerom and sweet Basil of each an oz., of cloves 2 oz., yellow Sanders 2 oz., of Citron pills 7 drams, of Lignum Aloes 1 oz., of Benjamin 1 oz., of Storax 1 oz., of Musk 1 dram; bruise all these, and put them into a bag of silk or linnen, but silk is the best. [There is a note about measurements on p. 36.]

Gervase Markham,
The English Huswife, 1625

Lavender Sachet – Nineteenth Century

16 cups ground lavender
   flowers
120 g (4 oz.) gum benzoin
   in powdered form

7 ml (¼ fl. oz.) attar
   of lavender

Lavender Sachet, 1880

4 cups dried thyme
4 cups dried lemon thyme
4 cups dried mint
4 cups dried marjoram
8 cups dried lavender

8 cups dried rose heels (white
   base of petal removed)
⅔ cup ground cloves
5 cups dried calamus root
Scant 2 g ($\frac{1}{16}$ oz.) grains
   of musk

Modern sachets are less complex. Here are some recipes I like; the fragrances are generally light, but last well. I make small muslin bags, or flat muslin envelopes, depending on the end use of the sachets, and decorate them with a length of narrow satin ribbon; for gifts, I add a dried rosebud.

Rose Sachet

In this recipe the vetiver is used as a fixative; santal has a special affinity for rosebuds.

4 cups dried rosebuds
2 cups vetiver [p. 32]

4 tablespoons ground santal
   (sometimes called white or
   yellow sandalwood) or 8
   tablespoons sandalwood
   raspings

The vetiver comes in rootlike strands that should be pulled apart into smaller sections. Mix all ingredients and put into small cotton sachet bags.

Chypre Sachet

This has a woodsy, slightly exotic smell. If you cannot get patchouli leaves, increase the quantity of rosebuds to ⅝ cup, and add 3 drops of patchouli oil. (For vetiver, see p. 32.)

¼ cup mace (blade, if possible,
   otherwise ground)
⅓ cup patchouli leaves

½ cup rosebuds
¾ cup shredded vetiver root
½ cup oakmoss or vanilla pods

Combine mace, patchouli and rosebuds. Pull vetiver and oakmoss into small pieces and add to other ingredients.

Lavender–Rosemary Sachet

This makes 1 sachet. Enlarge proportions according to the desired number of sachets.

2 tablespoons lavender
2 tablespoons rosemary
10 whole cloves

¼ teaspoon powdered dry orange peel

Mix ingredients and put into sachet bag.

Mint Sachet

This makes 2 sachets; increase amounts according to desired number of bags.

2 tablespoons peppermint leaves
2 tablespoons lemon verbena

2 tablespoons lemon balm
2 tablespoons rosebuds

Mix all ingredients and put in sachet bag.

Sweet Bag to Perfume Linens

½ cup dried rosebuds
⅓ cup orris-root powder
1 cup coriander seeds, bruised in mortar

1 teaspoon ground cinnamon
10 slightly bruised whole cloves
½ cup dried orange flowers
½ teaspoon common salt

Mix well and fill small cotton bags.

Hanger Bags for Wardrobe

½ cup rosebuds
½ cup lavender

¼ cup thyme
Small stick cinnamon (about 12-mm or ½-inch), crushed

Mix and fill little bags and suspend on hangers in wardrobes to perfume clothes.

Dry-Scented Sachet

This fills 1 sachet. Increase amounts according to the number of sachets you want to make. This fragrance is particularly suitable for men.

2 tablespoons lavender   1 tablespoon lemon balm
2 tablespoons thyme

Mix ingredients and fill bags.

Perfumed Writing Paper

Use favourite sachet powder and fill tiny bags to slip in writing-paper box.

Perfumed Linen Papers

Place envelopes filled with sachet powder between stacked sheets of linen paper; cure together 6 weeks.

WASH BALLS

The custom of washing with perfumed soaps is as old as time, but there is a direct relationship between the medieval custom of dipping the hands into rose water after a meal and the later development of scented wash balls made with rose water and other lovely fragrances. Cleaning the hands after meals was a necessity – there were no forks. In the courts and in the homes of the nobility it was the custom to place a bowl of rose water on the dining table even in the dark years before the twelfth century. There's a record that in 1140, when Matilda, heiress to the English throne, was engaged to Geoffrey, Count of Anjou, she received as a gift from France a silver peacock set with precious stones and designed to hold rose water so guests could dip their hands in it after dinner.

We have such lovely perfumed soaps today that there's not much temptation to make your own. I've made soap from scratch with hardwood ashes and lamb fat. Try, if you like. The recipe goes about like this: sift 8 cups of ashes, keeping only the very fine. Put them into a crock and cover with boiling water. Allow to soak 10 days, then strain the water and save, and throw away the ashes. (The water feels soapy and is a potent cleaner.) Over a low heat, melt lamb fat to a medium low point. Stir in about half a cup of lye (which is what you have produced from the wood ashes), and let the mixture cool. Stir in perfume, pour into moulds, and let dry for several weeks. Balls of fern, burned until they 'become blewish', were used in the early days in England as a lye cake and dissolved in wash water for clothes.

A much easier way to make perfumed wash balls is given below. I use Ivory soap because it is soft when first unwrapped, and melts quickly in water. But any soap will do. The stillroom ladies usually made their perfumed wash balls with castile soap.

Wash Ball with Soap

A double bar soap   *3 drops lavender oil*
¼ cup rose water   *Rose water*

Slice the soap into thin strips; heat the rose water and pour it over the soap. Allow to set for 10 minutes, mix well, then turn into a blender, adding the lavender oil a drop at a time. Cool and pour into a small, round mould. When soap has set and begun to dry out – 2 or more days depending on the weather – scoop up and form into balls. Set in the sun to dry. When almost dry, moisten your hands with rose water and rub the wash ball between them until the surface is smooth and shiny.

If you want to try a stillroom wash ball, combine the soap recipe with instructions for these two stillroom 'receipts'. The recipes are from the *Receipt Book of Charles Carte*, Cook to the Duke of Argyll (1732).

Perfumed Wash Balls

Dissolve musk in sweet compounded Water, then take about the quantity of one Wash-ball of this Composition, and mix it together in a mortar. Mix this well with your Paste, and make it up into balls.

Delicate Wash Ball

Take four Ounces of the Flowers of Lavender, 4 ounces of Calamus Aromaticus, 2 ounces of Rose leaves, 2 ounces of Cypress, and 6 ounces of Orris; pound all these together in a Mortar, then searse [sieve] them through a fine searse, then having scrapped a sufficient quantity of Castile soap, dissolve it in Rose-Water, mix the Powder with them, beat and blend them well together in a Mortar, then make them into Balls.

POMANDERS AND SCENTED BEADS

The original pomander – *pomme d'ambre* – was a small apple-shaped lump of ambergris, a strongly scented fixative. In time the name, which is French for 'apple of ambergris', referred to the exquisite gold, silver, ivory, wood or crystal cases in which these fragrant balls were placed. Hung from necklaces or belts, the purpose of the pomander was to protect the wearer from foul smells and to avoid infection.

In the early days of England, tinkers carried bracelets and necklaces of perfumed gums, which were threaded together with lengths of string. Mary Doggett, our stillroom lady, recommends making them the size of a nutmeg and colouring them with lampblack. Elizabeth I usually carried a pomander made in the shape of a ball and composed of benzoin and ambergris. She also owned 'a faire gyrdle of pomanders'. Mary, Queen of Scots, owned a similar pomander, still displayed at Holyrood House in Edinburgh; it is all silver and was hung from her belt by a silver chain.

The pomander we can buy commercially today, a china ball perforated with small holes and filled with fragrant herbs, is a replica of an earlier type of pomander and can be seen in an illustration published in 1502 in *Boat of Foolish Women* by Jodocus Badius.

The pomander most commonly made for Christmas giving, an orange stuck with cloves, is similar to the one Cardinal Wolsey used – on visiting days he carried it with him tied to his belt to keep away the evil odour of the streets and of his parishioners.

Pomanders made of citrus fruits stuck with cloves are easy to make as long as you wear a thimble on the thumb that does most of the clove-pushing. They are always welcome holiday gifts. We make them three weeks before Christmas, and wrap them in muslin, then in a big square of red or green netting tied with gold ribbons and tiny Christmas bells. Piled in a big silver bowl close to the front door, they are very festive, and as our guests depart we give each one a pomander. The fragrance of a citrus pomander kept closed in a drawer is cloves-plus, a spicy scent that holds for years.

Modern Citrus Pomander

Allow yourself a week to punch all the cloves into the fruit. If your thumb gets sore, poke holes in the fruit with a knitting needle, then press the cloves into the holes.

1 orange, lemon, or *lime*	*About 30 g (1 oz.) whole*
4 tablespoons orris-root powder	*cloves*

Punch cloves into the fruit so close together they touch. Put the clove-scented fruit into a mixing bowl, and sift over it the orris-root powder; scoop up and pour the powder until the fruit is completely coated white. Place it in a brown paper bag and set it away in a dark cupboard to dry out and ripen. Wrap first in muslin, to keep the orris-root from brushing off, then in another prettier wrapper for giving. In time the pomander will become completely dry and can be unwrapped if you want to wear it as the Elizabethans did.

A small pomander attached to a string makes a fascinating traditional gift. In earlier times, pomanders were made of precious gums and resins, of myrrh and spikenard, as well as ambergris, and included the fixatives benzoin, storax, civet, and musk. The core of less costly pomanders was plain garden soil or gumdragon, which is the dried resin of a species of *Astragalus*. This swells and jells in water. Gumdragon is used as an emulsifier and as a thickening agent for pills.

Here are some recipes from long ago. Since musk grain is difficult to get and very costly, the chances are you'll have to work out substitutes for some of the ingredients here. Some early recipes direct us to beat damask rose petals to a paste and use that as a base; certainly this will be less perfumed (and less expensive) than musk. p. 36 advises on measures.

Eighteenth-century Beads

Take Benjamin, Labdanum and Storax of each an ounce. Then heat a mortar very hot and beat them all to a perfect paste adding four grains of Civet and six of musk. Then roll your paste into small beads, make holes in them and string them while they are hot.

John Middleton,
Receipt Book, 1734

Perfumed Necklace

One oz. of Benjamin, 1 oz. of Storax and 1 oz. of Labdanum. Heat in a mortar very hot, and beat all these gums to a perfect paste; in beating of it, put in 6 grains of Musk, 4 grains of Civet. When you have beaten all this to a fine paste, wet your hands with rose water, roll it round betwixt your hands, and make holes in the beads, and so string them while they be hot.

C. J. S. Thompson,
The Mystery and Lure of Perfume, 1927

Mary Doggett's Pomander

Take a quarter of an ounce of civit, a quarter and a half-quarter of an ounce of Ambergreese, not half a quarter of an ounce of ye spiritt of Roses, 7 ounces of Benjamin, almost a pound of Damask Rose buds cut. Lay gumdragon in rose water and with it make your pomander, with beads as big as nutmegs and color them with Lamb [sic] black; when you make them up wash your hands with oyle of Jasmin to smooth them, then make them have a gloss, this quantity will make seaven Bracelets.

Mary Doggett,
Her Book of Recipes, 1682

The following paste was used by the Duchess of Braganza and the Duchess of Parma in the late sixteenth century. A cassolette is a small box with a perforated lid through which the scent was sniffed.

Paste for a Cassolette

Ambergris 3 drachmas, musk 2 drachmas, civet 1 drachma, essence of citron 3 drachmas. Mix the ambergris, musk and civet together, then add the oil and essence and make the whole into a paste with rose-water and place in the cassolette.

C. J. S. Thompson,
The Mystery and Lure of Perfume, 1927

Pomander – Sixteenth Century

Take 2 oz. of Labdanum, of Benjamin and Storax, 1 oz.; musk, 6 graines; civet, 6 graines; Ambergrease, 6 graines; of Calamus Aromaticus and Lignum Aloes, of each the weight of a groat; beat all these in a hot mortar, and with a hot pestall till they come to paste; then wet your hands with Rose-water and rowle up the paste suddenly.

Sir Hugh Platt,
Delights for Ladies, 1594

The following instructions for bringing life back to a fading pomander are from Ram's *Little Dadoen* (1606).

To Renew the Scent of a Pomander

Take one grain of Civet, and two of Musk, or if you double the proportion, it will bee so much sweeter; grinde them upon a stone with a little Rose-water; and after wetting your hands with Rose-water you may worke the same in your Pomander. This is a sleight to passe away an old Pomander; but my intention is honest.

TO KEEP MOTHS AWAY

From earliest medieval times, housewives concocted sweet-smelling herb bags to protect their linens and woollens against moths and other damaging insects. Specific herbs were grown in the garden for just this purpose. In *Banckes's Herbal*, published in 1525, Richard Banckes mentions rosemary: 'Also take the flowres and put them in a chest amonge your clothes or amonge bokes and moughtes [moths] shall not hurte them.'

Rosemary was used by the German housewife against all kinds of vermin, and the French so trusted rue and southern-wood that they called both the herbs 'garde robe'. The Pennsylvanians used southernwood to keep moths and ants from their closets. A less common herb, lavender cotton, *Santolina chamaecyparissus*, was cultivated in colonial days, along with woodruff, to keep moths from woollens. Lavender is considered a moth deterrent too. In India, vetiver is used.

In addition to keeping moths away, most herb bags had a second purpose; they perfumed drawers and closets and the recipes included materials meant to give fragrance as well as protection. But the moth bag isn't the same as a sachet, whose sole purpose is to perfume. The recipe below is American, from the nineteenth century, and comes from *The Practical Housewife*, published in 1860.

Moth Bag

Take of cloves, caraway seeds, nutmegs, mace, cinnamon and tonquin beans, of each 1 oz. [30 grammes]; then add as much

Florentine orrisroot as will equal the other ingredients put together. Grind the whole well to powder, and then put it in little bags, among your clothes.

Sweet Bag against Moths

This is an adaptation of an old European recipe for a sweet bag to keep moths away – it has an exquisite fragrance. Place mixture in small squares of muslin edged with ribbon, or into ribbon-edged muslin triangles. If you cannot obtain cedar powder, try adding an extra cupful of dried lavender flowers and about $\frac{1}{4}$ cup of cedar fragrance. You can leave out the cedar altogether without destroying the bag's moth-proofing properties.

$\frac{2}{3}$ cup orris-root powder
2 cups loosely packed shredded
    vetiver root
$\frac{2}{3}$ cup ground cloves

2 cups dried rose petals
2 cups dried lavender flowers
1 cup cedar powder
4 drops oil of roses

Combine all ingredients except the rose oil. Add the rose oil drop by drop, mixing well. Seal into a plastic bag and cure for 2 weeks. Pour into small muslin bags and tie with rose or lavender ribbon.

The French Recipe

This adaptation of an old French recipe against moths includes many fragrant herbs.

1 cup dried rosemary
1 cup dried tansy
1 cup dried thyme

1 cup dried mint
1 cup southernwood
$\frac{1}{2}$ cup ground cloves

Chop and mince all the herbs together and mix with the cloves. Pour into little muslin bags and tie with coloured ribbon.

Cape Cod Moth Repellent

This is a modern anti-moth preparation that really works.

3 cups dried moneywort   3 cups dried santolina
3 cups dried tansy

Chop together, mix well, place in muslin bags tied with ribbons.

Here are three fragrant herbal moth repellents that make charming and inexpensive little gifts.

Herbal Moth Bags

This fills two moth bags.

¼ cup dried, crumbled tansy   ¼ cup dried thyme
¼ cup dried mint   1 tablespoon crushed
¼ cup dried wormwood   cinnamon stick

Mix ingredients, put in muslin bags, and store among clothes.

Southernwood Moth Bags

This is enough for one bag; increase proportions according to number needed.

2 tablespoons dried lavender   1 tablespoon dried
1 tablespoon dried rosebuds   southernwood

Combine ingredients and place in small muslin bags tied with ribbons.

French Southernwood Moth Bag

This is enough for one bag; increase according to the number needed. The herbs are dried (p. 57).

3 tablespoons southernwood	*2 tablespoons tansy*
2 tablespoons thyme	*1 teaspoon ground cloves*

Combine and pour into small muslin bags tied with ribbon.

TO PERFUME LINENS

Although one purpose for sachets and sweet bags was to guard against moths, the stillroom ladies also used them to perfume linens. Sometimes it is difficult to distinguish between moth bags and sweet bags in old herbals and cookbooks.

Pot marjoram (*Marjorama onites*) was a good herb for scenting linens, but from the early 1500s lavender was the most popular of all scents for this purpose. The expression, 'laid up in lavender' probably dates from that period. 'Let's go to that house,' says English writer Izaak Walton in the seventeenth century, 'for the linen looks white and smells of lavender and I long to be in a pair of sheets that smell so.' The romantic poet John Keats refers to lavender in his 'Eve of Saint Agnes' (1819):

> And still she slept an azure-lidded sleep,
> In blanched linen, smooth, and lavender'd.

There were, of course, other sixteenth-century favourite scents and royalty has left records of their preferences. Elizabeth I liked sandalwood both for her linens and her clothes. King Henry of France used violet powder. His special recipe included 'orris root, rose leaves, santal wood, chypres, benjamen, marjoleine, storax, calamus, giroffle, ambergris, coriander and lavender'. The fifteenth-century English king Edward IV had his things scented with anise and orris powder and has left a record of his preference in 1480 wardrobe accounts. Queen Isabella of Spain's favourite, listed in 1631, contained rose leaves and 'calamus, girofle flowers, orris, storax, coriander'.

There are simpler ways to perfume linen. In Sicily, the women still dry the newly washed clothes on lavender and rosemary bushes. You can make simple sachets by stuffing little bags with any of these: rose leaves scented with patchouli oil (about three drops to every third of a cup), ground tonka beans, fresh woodruff, dried costmary (this is the culinary herb *Chrysanthemum balsamita*) mixed half-and-half with lavender, orris-root powder with a few drops of rose oil mixed in, and, of course, everyone's standby, lavender.

Dear old Sir Hugh Platt, in his *Delights for Ladies* (1594), has a scented water to sprinkle over dry clothes when they are being moistened for ironing – or so I understand his strange title:

To make a special sweet water to perfume clothes in the folding being washed. Take a quart of Damaske-Rose-Water and put it into a glasse, put unto it a handful of Lavender Flowers, two ounces of Orris, a dram of Muske, the weight of four pence of Amber-greece [ambergris], as much Civet, foure drops of Oyle of Clove, stop this close, and set it in the Sunne a fortnight: put one spoonfull of this Water into a bason of common water and put it into a glasse and so sprinkle your clothes therewith in your folding: the dregs, left in the bottome (when the water is spent) will make as much more, if you keepe them, and put fresh Rose water to it.

In the most recent edition (1969) of *Yorkshire Cooking*, compiled and edited by Shirley Kate of the Halifax Courier Ltd, there's a recipe for perfuming linen. An adaptation of it suitable for the harvest of our gardens relies on the availability of fragrant rose petals:

Dry Perfume for Linens

If your rose petals are not the highly fragrant kind, use any colourful dried rose petals, and add 8 drops of oil of roses to the recipe. Mix extremely well with other ingredients, seal and cure, shaking daily, before using. This recipe fills 24 tiny linen bags.

16 cups dried rose petals	⅓ cup cinnamon, ground
⅓ cup cloves, ground	8 tonka beans, chopped
⅓ cup mace, ground	2 cups orris-root powder
⅓ cup caraway seeds, ground	

Chop all ingredients together into a mealy powder; then put the mixture into little bags and lay among the linens.

Perfumed Starch

This recipe, adapted from the days of Tudor England's great lacy collars and ruffs, is easy to reproduce. If your roses are not fragrant, add 4 drops of rose oil before adding the musk.

4 cups fragrant rose petals	8 cups boiling water
2 cups fresh lavender flowers	4 drops oil of musk or
1 cup fresh rosemary	ambergris
1 cup sage	Dry starch

Mash everything but the water, oil and starch. Turn the mashed ingredients into a wide saucepan with the boiling water. Simmer, covered, until the water has reduced and thickened. Let the liquid cool, drop in oil, cover, and let stand overnight. Strain and bottle. Add lumps of dry starch to this mixture as directed on the starch package.

Here are three more recipes to investigate from the sixteenth and eighteenth centuries. (Rose 'leaves' here mean petals.)

Eighteenth-century Bags for Linen

[Rhodium is rosewood. Use rose oil as a substitute.]

Eight oz. of coriander seeds, 8 oz. sweet orris root, 8 oz. damask rose leaves, 8 oz. calamus aromaticus, 1 oz. mace, 1 oz. cinnamon,

½ oz. cloves, 4 drachms musk powder, 2 drachms white loaf sugar, 3 oz. lavender flowers, and some of Rhodium wood, beat them well together and make them in small silk bags.

Hannah Glasse,
The Art of Cookery, 1747

Sixteenth-century Sweet Water for Linens

Three pounds of Rose water, cloves, cinnamon, Sauders [sandalwood], 2 handfull of the flowers of Lavender, lette it stand a moneth to still in the sonne, well closed in a glasse; Then destill it in Balneo Marial. It is marvellous pleasant in savour, a water of wondrous swetenes, for the bedde, whereby the whole place, shall have a most pleasaunt scent.

Bulleins Bulwarke, 1562

To Make Swete Powder for Bagges

Take Damask rose leaves, orrisroot, calaminth, benzoin gum and make into a powder and fill ye bagges.

C. J. S. Thompson,
The Mystery and Lure of Perfume, 1927

SCENTED INKS

In the days when manor houses were equipped with morning rooms and ladies had enough leisure time to sit in them and attend to social correspondence, paper and envelopes and pens were beautiful affairs, and inks were often scented. Perfumed ink has a very faint fragrance but it is strong enough to be noticeable when an envelope is opened, and the scent lingers. You can make your own scented ink from any strongly aromatic herb. Delicately fragrant herbs don't boil down to a solution strong enough to mask the scent of the ink itself, so use dried herbs, preferably herb tips picked just before the buds open.

Lemon Verbena Ink

½ cup tightly packed lemon verbena	1 bottle ink (about 2 fl. oz., or 56 ml)
½ cup water	

Crush the verbena leaves, and place in a small enamel saucepan with the water. Bring to a boil rapidly, then simmer covered for 45 minutes to 1 hour. Watch out that the water boils down but does not evaporate completely. The scent is ready when the water is brown and opaque. Strain the liquid into a cup, discard the leaves. To 1 bottle of ink add 3 to 4 teaspoons of the herb liquid. The potency of the scent will vary according to the quality of the dried herb.

Rosemary Ink

¼ cup rosemary	1 bottle ink
⅓ cup water	

Follow the directions for Lemon Verbena ink, but reduce the simmering time to 30 minutes.

SCENTED CANDLES

Scented candles are associated with religion, and they date back to classical Rome, but it is the New World that has given us some of the best materials for making fragrant candles.

The first Christian Emperor of Rome, Constantine the Great, built the first church of Christendom, Saint-John-in-Lateran, and provided scented wax candles to be burned continually. When Clovis, the first Christian king of France, was baptised in Reims on Christmas Day, 496, fragrant tapers were lit and held by those who attended. Perfumed candles were also burned in most upper-class homes in Georgian England two centuries ago, and they were usually set in cut-glass fixtures.

Early settlers in America made ample use of wax myrtle, a shrub found on the wastelands of Nova Scotia and as far south as Louisiana. *Myrica cerifera* was commonly called the candle-berry, and night lights were made from the white wax crust of the berries. To make the candles, the Colonials scalded the berries with boiling rain water and collected the wax as it floated to the surface. The yellow tallow was then reheated and made into cakes which burned with a smokeless clear white flame that gave off an aromatic scent. The Indians obtained a fragrant wax from *Myrica gale*, the sweet gale, a native British plant widely spread through North America. The leaves yield an aromatic oil when distilled, and the small yellowish-green berries give a brittle wax which can be collected by the boiling water treatment. The wax when burned gives a delightful balsamic odour.

Candlemaking took place in November or early December in the South, just after the first heavy frost, which is when the waste fat from which candles were made is produced. The fat was boiled, caked, pressed, sieved and purified several times, and cotton wicks were inserted. (A finer-spun wick was made from milkweed.)

Bayberry (*Myrica pensylvanica*) candles were also made at about this time too, when the berries were ripest. So precious were the bayberry candles to the colonist that a fine was levied on anyone who picked the berries before autumn. With their waxy coat, they were thrown into a pot of boiling water, and when the wax floated to the top it was skimmed and cooled in moulds. In the 1700s the bayberry stood for Christmas, and the burning of a bayberry candle was as traditional in America as the yule log in England. The perfume of the snuffed berry was part of the magic of Christmas Eve.

Today we make our fragrant candles from ordinary candle wax, to which is added an essential oil. Among the nicest fragrances for scenting candles are bayberry, pine, lemon, gardenia, piñon pine (my own favourite), sandalwood, saddle leather, and frangipani. Honeysuckle, heliotrope and violet can be used in candles, too, but I find them too sweet for my taste. To make candles with these scents, follow the basic recipe for a Bayberry Night Light given below.

You can also combine several scents in one candle and come up with a unique perfume. In 1639 Philibert Guibert, Physician Regent of Paris, in his book, *The Charitable Physician* (1639), gave these instructions:

Scented Candle

[Gum dragant was a substance also known as gumdragon which jelled in water and was here used as a jelling agent.]

Take Benjamin, Storax, of each foure oz., Frankincense, Olibanum, of each 12 oz., Labdanum 18 oz., Nigela, 1 oz., coriander seeds, Juniper berries, of each halfe an oz.; liquid Storax sixe oz., turpentine half an oz., form them into candles with gum dragant and Rose water.

You can make candles from materials and kits sold in craft and candle shops. The address of Candle Makers Supplies, a mail order firm, is given on p. 125. Stearic acid, mentioned in my basic recipe, is a desirable additive that makes the candle wax more receptive to colour and also makes it burn more slowly. To make scented candles, add some drops of essence.

Here is a basic recipe:

Bayberry Night Light

The fragrance of bayberry candles is most noticeable just after the wick has been snuffed out.

1 small tin to serve as the mould – a 7-oz. (200-g) orange-juice tin would do

225-g (½-lb.) block paraffin wax

1½ teaspoons stearic acid

1 teaspoon blue colour concentrate or 1 or more wax crayons

30 drops bayberry essence

125-mm (5-inch) piece candle wicking

Make a small hole for the wick in the bottom of the can. Oil it inside. Over *low* heat, melt the wax in a small saucepan; if you overheat, it may catch fire. Melting time is about 10 minutes. When the wax has melted, add the stearic acid, and when this has melted, add colour. To test colour, drop $\frac{1}{2}$ teaspoon of wax into cold water. The finished candle will be more opaque and therefore darker, than the sample. If you find the colour too pale, add more.

Remove the wax from the heat, and add the bayberry or other essence with an eyedropper. Dip the wicking in melted wax, pull taut and hold till the wax sets. Insert the waxed wick into the hole in the can, letting about $\frac{1}{4}$-inch of wick protrude from the other side. Attach this piece to the underside of the can with sticky tape. Make sure the tape is firmly secured to prevent wax from leaking. Pour the melted wax into the can and steady the wick with your other hand so it is central. Pour to within 6 millimetres ($\frac{1}{4}$ inch) from the top. Don't let the wax cool to the point where it starts to scum before pouring. If this should happen, reheat slightly and hold the wick in position between two barbecue skewers or two pencils while the candle sets.

In about 3 hours the wax will have cooled. Remove the tape, run a thin knife around the inside of the can, invert the can, and shake. If the candle doesn't come out easily, dip it in hot water briefly and try again. Clip the wick to the desired length. The candle will have an irregular surface which can be left as it is or polished with an old nylon stocking dipped in vegetable oil.

To clean the saucepans, run very hot water in them before scouring.

7
What to Grow

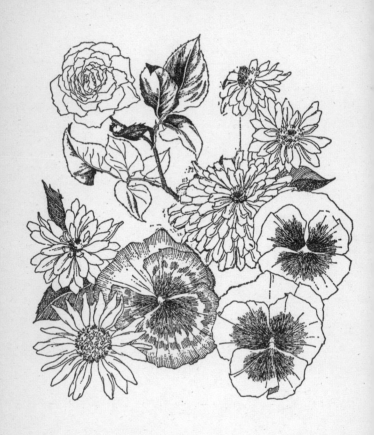

7

WHAT TO GROW

ONCE upon a time, many flowers were smaller and more fragrant than those we have today; herbs of all kinds grew in gardens; and tinkers and shadowy apothecary shops sold the fixatives and the gums, resins and spices with which the still-room ladies made their fragrant potpourris and pomanders. Today, we have fewer heavily scented flowers and it can be difficult to find the fixatives and fragrant oils that replace fragrant blossoms. Happily, garden centres, shops for the herb enthusiast and a few mail-order houses do their best to supply the materials needed to make the old fragrances (pp. 125–6).

A: OLD ROSES WITH FRAGRANCE

Two or three plants from this list will yield quantities of blossoms for your potpourri.

'Belle Poitevine': rugosa, lilac-pink
'Celsiana': damask, pink to blush
Common Moss: cabbage, pink
'Frau Dagmar Hastrup': rugosa, pink
'General Jacqueminot': hybrid perpetual, crimson
'Hansa': rugosa, cerise
'Reine des Violettes': hybrid perpetual, pink-purple
'Rose de Resht': autumn damask, fuchsia-red

B: FRAGRANT ROSES OF TODAY

'Crimson Glory': hybrid tea, red
Climbing 'Crimson Glory'
'Don Juan': large-flowered climber, red
'Etoile De Holland': hybrid tea, red

'Fragrant Cloud': hybrid tea, orange-red
'Helen Traubel': hybrid tea, pink
'Mirandy': hybrid tea, red
'Mr Lincoln': hybrid tea, red
'Sweet Fairy': miniature, pink
'Talisman': hybrid tea, orange-rose multicolour
'The Doctor': hybrid tea, pink
'Tiffany': hybrid tea, pink

C: OTHER FRAGRANT FLOWERS

PERENNIALS

Acorus calamus – sweet flag
Asperula odorata – sweet woodruff
Centranthus ruber – red valerian
Cheiranthus cheiri – wallflower
Chrysanthemum balsamita – costmary
Convallaria majalis – lily-of-the-valley
Dianthus – all species
Epigaea repens – trailing arbutus
Lavandula officinalis – English lavender
Lilium auratum – lily
Lilium candidum – Madonna lily
Monarda pectinata – lemon mint
Nicotiana alata – flowering tobacco
Rosa – many varieties (See Table A)
Valeriana officinalis – garden heliotrope, common valerian
Verbena teucrioides
Viola blanda – sweet white violet
Viola odorata – sweet violet

ANNUALS

Abronia umbellata – prostrate sand verbena
Asperula orientalis – Oriental woodruff

Datura meteloides – Hindu Datura
Heliotropium peruvianum – heliotrope
Lathyrus odoratus – sweet-pea
Matthiola bicornis – night-scented stock
Mimulus moschatus – musk flower
Reseda odorata – mignonette
Verbena hybrida – garden verbena

D: HERBS FOR THE STILLROOM

Here are some of the herbs often used for the old stillroom scents, antiseptics, cosmetics, and medicines.

ANNUAL

Anise – *Pimpinella anisum*
Basil – *Ocimum basilicum*
Borage – *Borago officinalis*
Chervil – *Anthriscus cerefolium*
Coriander – *Coriandrum sativum*
Cumin – *Cuminum cyminum*
Dill – *Anethum graveolens*

Heliotrope, garden – *Valeriana officinalis*
Nasturtium – *Tropaeolum majus*
Pennyroyal – *Mentha pulegium* (British); *Hedeoma pulegioides* (American)
Pot-Marigold – *Calendula officinalis*

BIENNIAL

Alkanet – *Anchusa officinalis*
Angelica – *Angelica archangelica*

Caraway – *Carum carvi*
Clary – *Salvia sclarea*

PERENNIAL

Alkanet – *Anchusa officinalis*
Balm, lemon – *Melissa officinalis*
Bay – *Laurus nobilis*

Bedstraw, Lady's – *Galium verum*
Burnet – *Sanguisorba officinalis*
Cardamom – *Amomum cardamon*
Chamomile – *Anthemis nobilis*
Costmary – *Chrysanthemum balsamita*
Elecampane – *Inula helenium*
Geranium, lemon and rose – *Pelargonium* (various species)
Hyssop – *Hyssopus officinalis*
Lavender – *Lavandula officinalis*
Lavender cotton – *Santolina chamaecyparisus*
Lemon verbena – *Lippia citriodora*
Lovage – *Ligusticum scoticum*
Marjoram, sweet, or knotted – *Origanum majorana*
Mint – *Mentha* (various species)
Peppermint – *Mentha piperita*
Rosemary – *Rosmarinus officinalis*
Rue – *Ruta graveolens*
Sage – *Salvia officinalis*
Southernwood – *Artemisia abrotanum*
Spearmint – *Mentha spicata*
Tansy – *Chrysanthemum vulgare*
Tarragon – *Artemisia dracunculus*
Thyme – *Thymus vulgaris*
Thyme, lemon – *Thymus citriodorus*
Woodruff, sweet – *Galium odoratum*
Wormwood – *Artemisia absinthium*

E: FLOWERS TO DRY FOR COLOUR

These flowers dry well and can be used to bulk out and to give additional texture and colour to potpourris and other dry perfumes.

Baby's breath
Blue and red salvia
Cockscomb
Goldenrod

Statice
Yarrow
Pansy
Hydrangea

Acacia
Heather
Pussy willow
Marigolds
Zinnias
Delphinium
Larkspur

Clematis
Black-eyed Susan
Queen Anne's lace
Scarlet sage
Celosia
Forget-me-nots

F: LANGUAGE OF THE PLANTS

Here are some of the meanings attached to flowers and herbs
in the Elizabethan and later centuries.

Angelica – soaring thoughts
Balm – compassion
Basil – love
Borage – courage
Burnet – gaiety
Chamomile – meekness,
        patience
Columbines – unchastity
Coriander – merit
Cumin – fidelity
Daisy – wantonness,
        faithlessness
Elder – sympathy
Fennel – flattery, dissembling
Forget-me-not – faithfulness
Heartsease – remembrance
Heliotrope – eternal love
Hyssop – sacrifice
Larkspur – infidelity
Bay laurel – glory
Lavender – silence

Lily – purity
Lily-of-the-valley – purity
Marigolds – happiness,
        remembrance
Marjoram – happiness
Mint – wisdom
Nasturtium – patriotism
Pansies – love, courtship
Parsley – rejoice
Pennyroyal – escape
Pimpernel – a meeting
Clove pink – resignation
Red rose – love
Hundred-leaved rose – grace
Musk rose – capricious
        beauty
White rose – silence
Yellow rose – infidelity
Rosemary – remembrance
Rue – repentance, grief
Saffron – joy, laughter

SOURCES

HERE is a list of reliable sources for materials. Many health food shops now also stock herbs, spices and some other ingredients. Chemists often carry essential oils, of varying strength and quality.

Culpeper Limited
  21 Bruton Street, London, WIX 7DA
  9 Flask Walk, Hampstead, London, NW3
  14 Bridewell Alley, Norwich, Norfolk

Herbs. Spices. Coarse sea salt. Perfumes and essential oils. Fixatives. Dried flowers and leaves. Potpourris, pomanders, etc. (Catalogue. Mail order from Hadstock Road, Linton, Cambridge.)

G. Baldwin & Co.
  173 Walworth Road, London, SE17 1RW

A particularly wide range of oils and floral essences. Fixatives, including myrrh and frankincense. Herbs, spices. Reasonable prices. (List of oils. Mail order.)

Caswell-Massy Co. Ltd
  320 West 13th Street, New York, N.Y. 10014, U.S.A.

Petals, herbs, fragrant woods. Fixatives. Tinctures of musk, ambergris and civet. Fragrant oils, including oakmoss and vetiver. (Catalogue. Mail order to Europe.)

Candle Makers Supplies
  4 Beaconsfield Terrace Road, London, W14 0PP

Supplies list. Mail order.

J. Floris Ltd
89 Jermyn Street, London, SW1Y 6JH

Potpourris, pomanders. A special potpourri reviver. (Catalogue.)

The following nurseries carry fragrant roses, and will probably be able to supply some, at any rate, of those mentioned in List A on p. 119:

Hillier & Sons
Romsey Road, Winchester, Hampshire

J.S. Mattock
Dolphins Rose Nurseries, Oxford

Murrells of Shrewsbury
Portland Nurseries, Oteley Road, Shrewsbury, Salop

Sunningdale Nurseries Ltd
Windlesham, Surrey

For herb plants and seeds, as well as dried herbs:

The Old Rectory Herb Garden
Rectory Lane, Ightham, Sevenoaks, Kent

Meadow Herbs Ltd
47 Morton Street, London, SW1

Essential oils, herbs and spices. Potpourris, pillows, cushions and sachets.

INDEX

MORE ABOUT PENGUINS
AND PELICANS

For further information about books available from Penguins please write to Dept EP, Penguin Books Ltd, Harmondsworth, Middlesex UB7 0DA.

In the U.S.A.: For a complete list of books available from Penguins in the United States write to Dept CS, Penguin Books, 625 Madison Avenue, New York, New York 10022.

In Canada: For a complete list of books available from Penguins in Canada write to Penguin Books Canada Ltd, 2801 John Street, Markham, Ontario L3R 1B4.

In Australia: For a complete list of books available from Penguins in Australia write to the Marketing Department, Penguin Books Australia Ltd, P.O. Box 257, Ringwood, Victoria 3134.

In New Zealand: For a complete list of books available from Penguins in New Zealand write to the Marketing Department, Penguin Books (N.Z.) Ltd, P.O. Box 4019, Auckland 10.

SIMPLE KNITTING

Maj-Britt Engström

Knitting is *easy*.

Basically, all you need to know is how to cast on, knit plain and cast off – and these instructions and more are given in *Simple Knitting*.

Choose from any number of yarns, needles, colours and sizes and make your own sweaters, mittens, socks, scarves, shawls and ponchos.

EVERYBODY'S KNITTING

Kirsten Hofstätter

A medley of assorted patterns for the whole family to knit.

Kirsten Hofstätter has included all sorts of ideas and variations for pullovers, hats, scarves and other items, and suggests a number of ways to liven up the garments with knitted-in fruits, flowers and animals.

THE PENGUIN BOOK
OF KNITTING

Pam Dawson

The Penguin Book of Knitting will be invaluable, both for the beginner and for the more experienced knitter.

Pam Dawson, of the BBC Television knitting series, has put together an expert guide to different stitches and techniques, together with an imaginative selection of patterns for men, women, children and babies.

SIMPLE CLOTHES
and how to make them

Kerstin Lokrantz

Here are clear, detailed instructions on how to make simple clothes for men, women and children.

Some of the garments are very traditional – an Algerian *djelleba,* an artist's smock, a kimono, an Eskimo parka. All of them are functional, extremely easy to make and hardwearing, and Kerstin Lokrantz has lots of ideas for their trimmings.

PLAY WITH A PURPOSE
FOR UNDER-SEVENS

E. M. Matterson

Play is more important than the name implies: from it young children are learning all the time. But they need the right material to work on and a little guidance.

In this book the author gathers together information about pre-school playgroups which has emerged in the last decade and suggests answers to some of the questions which have arisen.

LEARNING THROUGH PLAY

Jean Marzollo and Janice Lloyd

This is a book chock full of ideas for simple games, activities and experiments, designed to help children develop their minds and their bodies.

The games can be played anywhere and many of them are, in fact, an extension of everyday jobs at home. They are all simple, practical and inexpensive, and require the minimum of equipment. Above all, they are immense fun, offering the reader a delightful and useful aid to the business of child-rearing.

THE PAUPER'S HOMEMAKING BOOK

Jocasta Innes

The Pauper's Homemaking Book is concerned chiefly with the pleasure to be found in creating – with the cheapest of materials and tools – a home of one's own. Jocasta Innes's book is directed towards those people who are setting up home in earnest, who have lots of ideas and energy, and – after paying out mortgage or rent – almost no cash.

There are dozens of ideas here for turning a garret, cottage or modern semi into a home. Jocasta Innes's suggestions are inventive and original, intended to make any enviroment cheerful and comfortable rather than merely habitable, and they are, above all, cheap.

THE PAUPER'S COOKBOOK

Jocasta Innes

The author has assembled a wealth (or should it be a poverty?) of recipes for meals costing between ten and twenty pence per head. Her collection of international, racially mixed and classless dishes promises good home cooking at 'Joe's Cafe' prices.

and

HERBS, SPICES
AND FLAVOURINGS

Tom Stobart

In his introduction Tom Stobart states, 'It has once more become necessary to *think* about flavours', and in this fascinating book he has compiled an alphabet of nearly 400 different herbs, spices and flavourings found throughout the world, based on extensive notes which he made on his travels in 70 countries.

The author gives a detailed description of their native uses, as well as their origins, history, magical, medicinal and scientific uses, together with a careful assessment of the graduations in taste and intensity, and the effects of cooking, freezing, pickling and maturing on them. In addition Tom Stobart examines synthetic and harmful flavourings, the growing of herbs for culinary purposes, and clears up any confusions that the reader might have, for instance, about the plethora of cooking oils, onions, mints and other commodities that are on the market.

Each entry is carefully assigned its scientific, botanical, native and popular names, and *Herbs, Spices and Flavourings* is illustrated throughout with both black and white drawings and colour plates.

and

GRANDMOTHER'S SECRET
Her green guide to health

Jean Palaiseul

For thousands of years wild herbs and flowers formed the basis of natural cosmetics, natural remedies and natural preventives. Gradually these properties have lost their credence beside the magic synthetics of 'modern' medicine. Now, at last, we are beginning to take a new interest in what our grandmothers can teach us, and Jean Palaiseul has written a book which is a mine of information about the folk lore, history and modern application of over 150 herbs and flowers.

For example, he tells us that *Honeysuckle* is rich in salycylic acid – the essential ingredient of aspirin – and an infusion of the flowers is a reliable help in bronchial complaints. *Garlic*, too, can prove an indispensable shield against winter colds, and the Ancient Egyptians and Greeks believed that it gave extra strength – the Pharaohs insisting that the pyramid builders ate a clove every day.

Categorized in alphabetical order and copiously illustrated with beautiful line drawings, this guide to health from plants will prove a useful and unusual addition to the family medicine chest.